DATE DUE			
AG 19 '93			
MR 1 8 '94			
AP 5 '94			
SE 2 2 '94			
AP 2 8 '95			
MY 1 4 '97			
FEB 1 8 1998			

NORMA S. UPSON

When Someone You Love Is Dying

A FIRESIDE BOOK
PUBLISHED BY
SIMON & SCHUSTER

Copyright © 1986 by Norma Upson
All rights reserved
including the right of reproduction
in whole or in part in any form
A Fireside Book
Published by Simon & Schuster, Inc.
Simon & Schuster Building
Rockefeller Center
1230 Avenue of the Americas
New York, New York 10020
FIRESIDE and colophon are registered trademarks of
Simon & Schuster, Inc.
Designed by CAUBER
Manufactured in the United States of America
10 9 8 7 6 5 4 3 2 1

Library of Congress Cataloging in Publication Data

Upson, Norma S.
  When someone you love is dying.
  Includes index.
  1. Terminal care. I. Title.
R726.8.U67   1986   649'8   86-13038

ISBN: 0-671-61079-1

Acknowledgments

I would like to thank:

Jodeanne Bellant, M.D.
Joan Buel
LeRoy Colvin
Regina Denton
Dolores Cortsy
The Dorian Group of Seattle
Dornbecker's Children's Hospital
Karen Fredricksen—Shanti of Seattle
Gay Men's Health Crisis, N.Y.C.
Gay Rights National Lobby
Elise Goodman
Kathy Hunter
Beverly Kennedy
Joyce McFettridge
The Oregon Health Sciences University
Derry Ridgeway, M.D.
Herbert Schaffner
Shriners Hospital for Crippled Children
Lendon Smith, M.D.
Marilyn Smith
Margaret Summers
Linda Van Burnen, R.N.
Elleen, Terry and Tiffany Volersten
Wilda Welch
Whitman-Walker Clinic
Carole Winner, Ph.D.
and many others who helped me research and write this book.

Dedicated with love to Bob

Table of Contents

Introduction   9

Part One: You and Emotions, Changes, and Stress

Chapter 1: Why? 15
Chapter 2: Emotions 17
Chapter 3: Changes 27
Chapter 4: Stress 43
Chapter 5: Support Systems (Friends and Helpers) . . . 55

Part Two: Options for Care

Chapter 6: Doctors, Communication, and
Understanding 67
Chapter 7: Hospitals 75
Chapter 8: Convalescent/Nursing Homes 82
Chapter 9: Home Care 88
Chapter 10: Hospices 96
Chapter 11: Help for the Bills 101

Part Three: Legalities and Decisions

Chapter 12: Very Important Papers 105
Chapter 13: Memorial and Funeral Planning 131

Part Four: Special Considerations

Chapter 14: Making Visiting Easier 141
Chapter 15: Nontraditional Couples 147
Chapter 16: Care of the Elderly 153

Chapter 17: Children 161

Afterword 167

Appendix I 169
Appendix II 182
Appendix III 202

Index 213

Introduction

"A man's dying is more the survivor's affair than his own."

—*Thomas Mann*
The Magic Mountain

For each terminally ill person, several more suffer a deep sense of loss, fear, guilt, frustration and stress. At a time when we most need support and counseling to deal with physical, emotional, spiritual and financial distresses brought about by the final illness of a loved one, we find we have neither time, energy nor resources to seek the help we need in order to put our life and situation in perspective.

When I became aware my husband was dying and there was no way I could alter the course of his illness, I found good and informative books which helped me understand somewhat the pattern and problems that imminent death might bring to him. But there was nothing and no one to guide *me* through the conflicts and turmoil within *me*.

Bob and I had always been together. As children we shared the swings and sandboxes of our neighborhood. We attended the same dancing and Sunday schools. We played tag as kids and post office in adolescence, and when we left home for school, we always kept in touch.

Married just before World War II, we weathered the problems of separation, GI educations, corporate mobility and raising our sons through the turbulent fifties and sixties. Now we were happily living together in a houseboat we had planned and built. We were looking forward to years of boating, fishing and travel. Instead, he developed a cough and the verdict was death in a few months.

Introduction

As devastating as that reality was, I could understand and even accept Bob's illness and death. I was not prepared, however, to understand and cope with something I had never experienced: my own deep-seated negative emotions. I was not equipped to make decisions by myself that Bob and I had always shared. I was angered by the medical terminology and my inability to persuade the doctor to discuss Bob's illness in anything but a clinical, perfunctory manner. I resented the feeling that I was intruding on hospital routine when I visited Bob. I could not make head or tail of the insurance forms and was half crazy with the ever-mounting bills not covered by hospitalization.

And there was *Guilt*. Voices inside me saying . . . "if I had only insisted that he do or not do something" . . . "perhaps I should have force-fed him vitamins, made him change doctors, prayed more fervently . . ." I was haunted by all the sins of omission and commission that collected over the years.

At first I could sail into the hospital with tokens of love and we'd share the day's happenings. We made his illness an adventure we could handle with humor and grace. We would fight together and beat the odds. But later, when there was no doubt this illness was terminal, the world came crashing in on me. We had been busy living; we had made no accommodation for death. Death was something that happened to other people. Now we were the other people.

This book is written for people like me who have not faced the intricacies, the taboos, the firestorms and the confusion terminal illness brings. It is a guide to those who are the supporting cast in the last act of a loved one's life. Hopefully it will shed some light on the daily mental, emotional, physical, spiritual and financial obstacles we experience as we approach the last good-bye.

While there are no pat answers for a person facing the loss of a loved one, there are certain similarities in the paths and patterns each of us experience during a terminal illness. There is comfort in knowing that the strange new emotions we feel are normal. It helps to know that what is happening to us has happened to others and can be shared. It is the sharing of those who have experienced a terminal illness as participants and care-givers that make up the information in this book.

Because it is written for *now*, when you are in the midst of tribulation, the book is brief. There are healthcare options, important legalities to consider and, I sincerely hope, there is comfort. The advice is from experienced people who have recently faced the decisions you are facing and from professionals who are dedicated to making this transition as comfortable as possible.

This is the book I needed when I struggled to make the best of the most difficult time of life, the time of farewell to the person I held most dear.

PART ONE

You and Emotions, Changes, and Stress

CHAPTER · 1

Why?

Ever since I began thinking there should be a guide for people who know someone they love is dying, I've been reading volumes of personal experiences and listening carefully to accounts of people going through the trials of a terminal illness. If there were any conclusions to be drawn, it is that there are no single answers for either the patients or survivors. But rich or poor, young or old, there are certain common factors everyone must face. You can be sure there will be emotional upheavals, there will be both subtle and drastic changes, and there will be stress.

I remember asking myself on a rare day of escape from the care of Bob: "What have I learned from all of this?" and the answer came back loud and clear: "I have learned that everything I thought I had learned from previous life experiences has changed or is changing. My faith, trusts, attitudes, values, relationships, fortitudes, self-regard, philosophy, appearance and even my dietary needs have changed or are changing. I scarcely recognize myself inside, and the outside of me is aging fast!"

This new person I was becoming was neither better nor worse so far as I could tell—only changed. I was no longer quite so certain of some things and I was far more certain of others. One thing I knew for sure is that *nothing* is for certain! On that day I adopted St. Thomas as my patron saint, for I understood with clarity why he answered his teacher, "Yes, Lord, I believe. Help thou my unbelief." I hope I will always remember what I now know—it is entirely human and understandable both to have faith and to question your beliefs as you try to bear up in a sea of fear, hurt and grief.

On that day I also realized that this was my private hell—a hell I found difficult to share with anyone. I decided I would have to ride out the storm of this torment by hanging onto whatever flotsam and jetsom of helpful philosophy and wisdom I could salvage from my life before it had become so difficult. Later, when the storm passed, I would have time to ask questions and seek answers.

Now it is later. I've spent the last five years exploring the turmoil I faced and which most of us face when we know someone we love is dying. I hope by exploring the common problems and experiences and sharing some solutions and answers, you will feel less alone and vulnerable.

Of great help (found out too late for me, but readily available to anyone who has a need) is the network of generous understanding people who willingly offer their experience and empathy so that you need not feel alone and helpless in your turmoil. I also found a very definite pattern in the way each of us responds to the coming death of a loved one, and so what we may *think* is an aberration may in fact be a perfectly normal response to the given situation. And it is crucial to truly understand that we cannot escape the death of a loved one and, eventually, our own death. This reality is harsh but in fact it's the key to living *now* with courage and strength and looking toward *later* with grace and assurance. Finally, you will learn, as I have, that nothing will ever be the same again, but life can and will flow on. You will be stronger and wiser for having lived life *now* to the best of your ability.

CHAPTER · 2

Emotions

Emotions, changes, and stress are the black trinity that will hound you from the time you realize your loved one is dying until long after the ordeal is over. How you cope depends on your character, background, personality, and an ability to adapt to changing situations.

The circle of emotion, stress, and change in all their varieties, orders and progressions speed faster and faster when your loved one is dying. Unless you recognize these symptoms and deal with them *as they occur*, you will be sucked into a vortex of helplessness and will lose the precious time you have left to be with the one you love.

The first emotion will most likely be *shock*. Shock takes many forms. My reaction was numbness. For days I lived in a kind of belljar, feeling nothing. I could see but could not touch or be touched. Then for a few weeks I was in a sort of daze where nothing made sense. What I felt is not unusual. The majority of people with whom I discussed my initial feelings about death confirm my belief that this sense of unreality and detachment is nature's way of preparing us for the onslaught of emotions to come.

There is not very much we can do for ourselves when we are in a deep phase of shock, but if friends and family as well as doctors recognize our condition and give us the time, space and support we need to recover, we will be stronger and better able to face coming difficulties.

During this period of shock you should not try to make important decisions quickly. Someone else should be given the responsibility of tending to normal, everyday chores and

stand by to help with plans and problems. Major decisions should be postponed. This is not a good time to expect yourself to be especially rational, stable, brave, philosophical, or devout. Those attributes will come at a later time. Now it is time to be totally self-caring and self-loving. If you allow yourself time to absorb the shock you will be better able to make proper decisions and understand what lies ahead.

People suffering from an emotional shock should be protected from the too readily available sleeping pills, drugs or liquor. The best medicine at this time is a hug, a comforting hand to hold, a cup of tea or soup, a small token of love and reassurance. Later, if stress becomes too great or if sleep becomes an elusive luxury, a doctor can prescribe something for relief. Most clinicians agree, though, that Nature's way is the best, allowing your realization to sink in gradually.

After the initial shock, it is not uncommon for a period of denial to strike. Denial comes in many forms and it is often shared by both a patient and his/her loved one. Many will flatly deny the illness. Many will be unable to register the information. Don't worry. It's perfectly normal to block out information in order to avoid the bitterness and confusion that accompany approaching death. This is what makes a support system so crucial now: you need people with better perspective to be on hand during the crisis (see "Doctors, Communication, and Understanding").

Another form of denial sends us running off in any direction to find someone, some medicine, some treatment to prove the diagnosis and prognosis were faulty and can be changed if only we find the right surgeon, shaman or healer. This is also normal. It is a natural temptation to think that if you can bundle your loved one off to a more acceptable place, there will surely be a cure.

Now, just when you're torn by denial and are trying to make sense out of the chaos around you, you may have the extra burden of family and friends who try to be helpful by advising you of new cures, marvelous healers, new procedures and discoveries. Expect to become vulnerable to many pressures from these well-meaning friends, but check out the opinions of the top specialists in your area before you become

involved in expensive, little-known and often hopeless treatments. If you hear of a miraculous cure, make it a point to *speak personally* to the cured person and ask to see his or her medical records.

There *are* alternative and viable means of treating diseases and there *are* ways and means of finding out what they are and who dispenses them. You would be remiss to blindly accept the first diagnosis without having other physicians and/or specialists confer about treatment; it is to that purpose I have included reference and resource materials at the end of this book. However, before you consider alternatives, it is important to find out exactly how the patient feels about changes and/or experimentations.

If your loved one resists the idea of going to a distant place or submitting to unusual therapies, it is wise and loving to respect these personal feelings, regardless of your desperation or high hopes. An adult who is desperately ill must have freedom of choice if he or she is to maintain the stamina, dignity and peace of mind necessary to bear up under stressful conditions.

At this point, when time, emotions and other resources are important considerations, it is far better to ask for second opinions, consultations and options within *known* boundaries than to shoot off on less proven tangents. When you have the opinions of the best specialists in the field, you can be certain that you have been given truth and the best advice. Stop there and consider it thoroughly with your loved one before going on.*

There will be guilt and uncertainty. There are always the haunting feelings that if you had insisted on checkups more regularly, if you had insisted on different behavior, if you had protected more, if you had or had not done this or that, he or she would not be ill. Few people losing a loved one do not feel pangs of guilt.

You must be rational. Can you honestly say you would

* *Center for Medical and Health Care Information, Inc., is one of the sources where one can find a critical evaluation of treatments and alternatives for medical consumers.*

knowingly act to hurt another? Should you accept the *total* responsibility of the actions or inactions of another? Who would not change something in the past if he or she could? The solution to deep guilt feelings is to force yourself to realize that you could not know all the causes and effects of life. You have done the very best you can. Stop whipping yourself.

If guilt becomes overwhelming, talk to a professional counselor. There are support groups, clergy, psychologists, doctors, mental health organizations and close friends who will help you bring these feelings of guilt into perspective (See also "Support Systems" and "Resources and Further Reading.")

Sometime during a long terminal illness you will become angry. It is natural to feel anger at care-givers, God, yourself and, most disconcerting of all, anger at the person who is ill. On the surface, these seem to be the targets of your anger, but you will realize that your anger is a natural manifestation of your frustration at the circumstances life has forced on you.

It is easy to say in a different setting, "We all must die" or "Death is a natural culmination of life" or "We are born, we live and die." But when death is close and personal and you feel the inevitable defeat of staving it off on a day-to-day basis, ponderous philosophic truths give little comfort and you may experience anger.

One of the most terrifying but common forms of anger is directed at the ill person. They may seem too submissive or radically changed in their personality. They may strike out against you and others closest to them. They may become sarcastic, uncooperative. They may become more dependent on friends or strangers than you like. You may feel isolated from or repulsed by them. Try to remember that the *illness* makes them selfish, indifferent, dull or hyperactive, demanding, morose, withdrawn, repulsive, or uncooperative. They may exhibit numerous other weird and unpleasant traits you never suspected were a part of their personality.

These phases of their illness and attitudes and your reactions to them are beautifully explained by Elizabeth Kubler-Ross in her book *On Death and Dying*. It is required reading for those who are facing the death of a loved one.

But what can *you* do about these mysterious changes and the anger they produce in you? Salvation comes by realizing that the changes (or what we perceive to be changes) are in *the illness, not the person.* Accepting changes of mood and behavior is the penalty we pay for loving and caring. This is not to say we should become doormats or martyrs; it is vital that the attending physician knows that drastic mood changes are taking place in the patient. And *your* anger and frustration should be discussed with understanding people. Your anger and frustration should also be discussed with the patient in a tolerant, rational way so that you and he/she understand that these are difficult times for *both* of you and that *both* of you must reach harmony and understanding if you are to cope.

Don't try to hide your anger and frustration. Vent it properly and honestly and you will find that because it *is* natural and normal, you can then deal with it without adding to the burden of guilt you'll feel during the after-death grieving process.

Sometimes medication causes a patient to become irritable or depressed. Occasionally the environment needs to be changed. Sometimes there is a need to bring in a third party who can communicate with the dying person and relay his or her feelings to others. There can be a multitude of reasons for the dying person's hurtful behavior. When *you* understand what is happening emotionally and spiritually to him/her, it makes it easier to cope with mood changes, unusual personality problems and with your own anger and frustration.

A friend who knew I was researching the effects of terminal illness on survivors asked, "Do other people struggle with the thought that perhaps smothering with a pillow or overdosing with medication would be far better than letting someone you love go on and on suffering—especially when you know they are going to die anyway?"

Of course they do. People faced with suffering have asked themselves and society this question throughout recorded history. Yet the dilemma is extremely personal and private. *Feeling* that you want to put a stop to the ordeal of suffering

21

is natural. But the *action* is irreversible and the consequences will have both a legal and psychological impact that can be devastating.*

At a time when medication and other procedures are available, suffering pain is not always necessary, nor is prolonging life beyond plausible limits. The Living Will† and a "No Code" on medical records clearly answer that problem. We are not gods, empowered to make life-and-death decisions for others, but doctors must be made to understand how both you and the patient stand on the issues of unnecessary pain and the prolongation of life beyond acceptable limits.

Is it natural to be repelled by the sights, smells and sounds of a desperately ill person whom you love with all your heart? Definitely. But always remember you are not repelled *by the person*—you are reacting to the indignities of dying. There are ways of ridding the room and bed of offensive odors by proper ventilation, deodorization, etc. and by insisting on good hygienic and grooming practices (barbers and hair stylists make home and hospital calls). And when groans, labored breathing, and mechanical sounds begin to tear at you, leave the room. Change *your* environment. I suggest getting a radio with headset attachments to escape any crazy-making noises.

As dearly as some of us would like to be saints, we may find we are offended by the sights, odors and sounds of illness, with its pipes, needles, thermometers, oxygen tanks and other paraphernalia. Overcoming these problems is both humiliating and challenging when you are the prime care-giver, but it *can* be done, by understanding the purpose of each article and apparatus. As for the odors, perhaps my experience with that part of care-giving will help.

The emotional responses we have to the sick room cannot be eliminated, but they can be understood. Bedpans, soiled linen and similar things have never been easy for me. I gag. I retch. I get *very* ill. When my nose is offended, my stomach

---

* *See p. 170.*
† *See p. 78.*

rebels. I can accept blood better than feces. God knows I've tried to overcome this weakness of character, but something in my stomach goes berserk when I'm confronted by bodily waste. With this in mind, you can imagine my consternation at the thought of being the only nurse during the last phase of my husband's illness. It shamed me but I was determined it wouldn't stand in the way of his last and greatest wish to be home.

I remember coming out of the bathroom one day shamefaced and still retching after emptying a bedpan. Bob took my hand and with his dry New England humor said, "Go ahead darling, gag and barf. Don't feel bad about it! The alternative to emptying that damned vessel could be devastating to both of us!"

It might not seem like much of a solution, but when I considered the alternatives, I knew he was right—he would either be back in a sterile hospital or he would not be *alive*. From then on, I knew I had chosen the right alternative. My stomach would rebel but I could carry on. I lost that anger at myself.

There will be anger and frustration with insurance companies, accounting departments, hospital/nursing facilities, friends, neighbors and associates. You will feel anger as everyone else's life sweeps by normally while yours is put on hold. You will be angry at what you perceive to be detachment by doctors and nurses.

Some days the whole world will be a target for your anger but hold your tongue and reason out *why* you are so angry. Remember that rectifying blunders you have made while in emotional turmoil is far more difficult than holding your tongue and giving others the benefit of the doubt.

Boredom is another problem you may have to deal with. Many of us become totally bored when we have to live on a daily basis with the long-term physical and mental limitations and disabilities of illness. Medical routines, visitations, lack of interest outside immediate pain or disability, and the humdrum expectations placed on you can become insupportably tedious. Everything is focused on the patient—nothing and no one else matters to him/her or the people involved in the care of the patient. *You* long to break away and think of something besides illness, death, care and giving. Don't fight it—*Get away!* Find something and someplace where you can forget your troubles for just a little while. Do something enjoyable and you will come back to sick room routines fresher and far more capable.

Sorrow, called pre-death grieving by experts, is another emotional bridge many of us must cross when we are dealing with the terminally ill. We equate bravery with stoicism and do not realize that one can be sorrowful and brave at the same time. It is healthy to give yourself permission to be sad and to express sorrow.

Why should we try to keep our loved ones from knowing we are sorry that they are gravely ill? Why should we not grieve that they are leaving us? To hide one's sorrow as if it was a dreadful secret or weakness can lead to all sorts of after-death grief problems.

Sharing sorrow with a loved one when there is to be a final parting can open doors and allow us to say things that are important at the time and vital to survivors after the beloved dies. We sometimes misconstrue sorrow as a weakness when in fact it is an honest tribute to the love we feel for each other.

Success in dealing with the terminally ill stems from understanding that your sorrow is natural. Your sorrow and mine at the thought of being left by the loved one is real and necessary if we are to look back at this time without regretting our omissions in sharing the sorrow of parting. Don't block emotions. Acknowledge them and deal with them. They are a natural form of love.

These are tried and true ways to help you through any emotional turmoil you are facing:

1. *Don't let things drift.* There are certain things that must be done, faced and put in order early in a terminal illness. Do them quickly and be done with them. If there are practical, business, or legal questions that must be answered, find out now

24

what they are and finalize them. *Ask* if there are wishes to be fulfilled, and take care of them *now*. If you are being questioned about the prognosis of the illness by the patient and loved ones, tell the truth. (See Part III, "Legalities and Decisions.")

2. *Make decisions.* If you need legal assistance or are in doubt about any of the practical, material aspects of policies, finances, indebtedness, property, etc., *get help immediately and make the necessary decisions* while the person who is ill is still capable of thinking rationally. (See "Legalities and Decisions.")

3. *Don't bottle up your fears.* Sort them out and find someone who can help you with them. (See "Support Systems.")

4. *Don't give in to guilt.* Don't blame others or yourself for past mistakes. The past cannot be changed. The present is all we can be sure we have. The future will come whether we want it or not. Take each day and make the best of it.

5. *Make your own life as comfortable as it can be.* Don't allow yourself to become a martyr—that's for saints. You and I are very real people with very real needs during these trying times. Treat yourself with kindness; it will bring both you and your loved one pleasure to know there are still some enjoyments in life.

6. *Don't play a role.* Be yourself and allow yourself to *be*. If you're frightened, worried or sorrowful, say "Help me." If you are being crowded, say "I need space. . . . I want to be alone for a while . . . I need a change of scenery . . . I need to cry." Enunciate your needs as they occur and they won't build up and overwhelm you. There are friends who will understand and supportive people who have experienced what you are feeling now—talk to them. (See "Support Systems.")

7. *Take care of yourself.* Eat wisely, get enough rest (you may not sleep, but bed rest can fill your

needs). Exercising in the fresh air is better than tranquilizers, but don't be too proud to accept medical help if it's needed. Take food supplements which will help your body deal with stress.

8. *Insist on your right to privacy.* Find a time and place where you can get away from telephone calls and other interruptions. Meditate, think, pray, read or listen to music and let your mind drift. Make this a time to rebuild inner strength—guard it zealously.

9. *Do something for others.* It's a mystery and a miracle that if you will look up from your own difficulties and help someone else in need, you will feel better. A few minutes of caring for or doing for someone outside your sphere of concern magically lightens your load.

10. *Make it a point to find at least three good things for which to be thankful for each day.* The longer the list, the better you will feel. Three blessings is the minimum.

11. *Memorize one short line* of a verse, proverb or wisdom which will bring you comfort. When things get tough, repeat the helpful quotation until you are in control. "This too shall pass" is a favorite of many.

12. *Look for humor.* Even black humor is better than none. There is someone or something out there that can make you laugh and forget for a minute that your life is grim—find it.

CHAPTER · *3*

Changes

Along with accepting the fact that there will be emotional storms during this time, we should also be prepared as best we can for the changes. For change is the only constant in terminal illness.

Changes that occur during this period can be shocking enough to give you nightmares or can be so subtle you will wonder if your imagination is playing tricks on you. Whatever the sign or symptom, change is stressful, emotional and inevitable and the sooner you can accept and adapt to the changes taking place in your loved one and in your world, the better you will be able to cope with the internal and external shifts taking place in our lives.

The fundamental need to adjust your attitudes, routines and expectations of yourself and others does not come easy, but it must come if you are to survive the firestorms and incapacities coming to you and your loved ones during this period.

The adapting or adjusting I speak of is not the worm-in-the-dust or go-with-the-flow passivity you may have experienced during shock. Instead you will evaluate and grasp what is happening and try to understand what you can and cannot do about your circumstances. The terminal illness of a loved one will be an exercise in endurance and you will learn to accept change as an important link between your emotional stability and your ability to coexist with stress.

The first and most difficult lesson is to accept that, while you cannot influence the devastating state of affairs in which you find yourself, *you can control your response to these situations.* When you have grasped the truth that you really do have choices within these hurtful and hateful circumstances, there is a surge of relief, and a sense of control and dignity that gives great inner strength at a time when you most need it.

You cannot be expected to have the detachment of the medical profession toward the illness but you can, with proper information, be prepared to handle the physical, mental and emotional erosions that come with most terminal illnesses.

A compassionate education by care-givers explaining what is and will be happening to the mind and body of the person who is ill removes some of the shock and prepares you emotionally. If you are prepared mentally, physically and spiritually to expect the degeneration common to most patients, you will have time to gather your resources, build your strength and face inevitable changes. Don't depend on the hearsay of friends and relatives. It is important that the side effects of medical and therapeutic treatments (positive as well as negative) be explained to you so that both you and the patient can make judgments based on an honest evaluation of your situation. You'll have to consider your respective philosophies, finances, capabilities, and temperaments.

It is your right and duty to obtain this medical and physical information just as it is your right and duty to make decisions with your loved one as to the kind of care and therapy to get. You *can* meet the changes and challenges if you are prepared. You *can* make the final days of life for your loved one more tranquil by accepting the changes you have known would take place. (See "Doctors, Communication, and Understanding.")

The changes I discuss briefly here are the most common and are the ones which should be explained to you more fully by competent professionals who are caring for your patient.

Among the first changes you can expect in your loved one are physical. It was no doubt physical symptoms (lump, blood, pain, mole, weakness, etc.) that sent him or her to the doctor in the first place. But now, the impact that this *is* a terminal illness, with all the grief and complications it implies, demands that you reassess your capabilities in order to determine how you can best direct your attitudes and actions to the long, trying period of physical erosion lying ahead.

It may be shocking to some that those who are being ripped apart by the diagnosis of a terminal illness can and should calculate and decide how to react to the diminishing strength and capabilities of a loved one. Yet in every case where survivors of a terminal illness (in hospice settings and/or home care) came through the ordeal successfully and in good emotional health, they mentioned that early in the illness they *consciously* made up their minds they could and would control the way *they* reacted to the physical aspects of the dying patient.

After the initial shock of diagnosis has worn away, it is time to make decisions about your life and the expectations of both you and the patient. Evaluate all physical changes *prior* to decision-making. *Now* is the time to decide who, if not you, will be the conduit for care and communication between the patient and the care-givers, financial and legal advisors. Remember to include the person who is ill in this process.

Physical changes not only encompass the altering condition of a patient's body but environmental changes as well. If John or Mary will not be able to climb stairs, make arrangements to accommodate that phase of his or her illness and control that problem in advance. Or, if you know eyesight will be increasingly impaired, find resources *now* for tools and entertainment for the sight-impaired. Environmental changes you make now can dovetail with the patient's expectations of physical changes, and it will become easier for both of you to accept. The changes you might expect to be made in the environment should be an important part of your discussions with the doctor, social worker or care-giver with whom you are dealing. (See "Doctors, Communication, and Understanding.")

The physical and sexual needs of the person you love will affect you deeply. Medication and/or disability often causes sexual indifference or impotence, which in turn causes stress and misunderstandings between people who have here-

29

tofore depended upon physical intimacy to strengthen them in crisis periods. Problems of this kind should be discussed with an understanding physician or therapist, someone with the expertise to guide you through sexual complexities which may seem hopelessly frustrating.

The physical changes which happen to you when you know someone you love is dying are only mentioned here but are more clearly delineated in the segments on emotion and stress. However, you should be aware of your own physical needs from the beginning of this illness until two or three years after it has been resolved.

I cannot emphasize too strongly the value of a physical checkup for *you*. You need to get the proper amount of sleep and nourishment, recreation and relaxation. *You* need to listen to your body and mind in order to adapt to inevitable changes.

There may be changes in a patient's personality. He or she may become bitter, hypercritical, jealous, frustrated, bored, selfish, indifferent, irritable, stubborn, angry, depressed, fearful, demanding, and perhaps even hysterical. The more you expect these changes, the better able you will be to cope with them. Emotional turmoil varies with the individual personality. There are no set times when they can be expected, but if you peg them as normal, natural behavior in the process, then you, your family, and the person who is dying will come through these difficult times with love intact.

There may be personality changes in a patient which are clearly and frighteningly *unnatural;* they should be discussed immediately with the doctor and/or care-givers. These changes can be an indication that something is radically wrong with medication, communication, or treatment. They can also be the natural pattern of the disease. Since you are the person most familiar with the personality and attitudes of your loved one, it is up to you to watch for and report these symptoms, and to insist they be reckoned with by your physician since his/her relationship with this patient has been of shorter duration, has been strictly on a professional level, or is dependent upon the reports of others.

Improper amounts or kinds of medication can bring about these problems and should be reported as soon as possible:

- Extreme highs—euphoric behavior which is out of touch with reality.
- Indifference to people and things which have always been important.
- Deep depression—a seemingly unresponsive attitude or an overly negative emotional response to everyday occurrences.
- Extreme nervousness—tremors, twitches, restlessness.
- Paranoia—suspicion of everyone's motives, fearful or evasive behavior.
- Extreme bitterness and sarcasm—unusually snide and nasty responses from a normally sweet-tempered person.
- Quick-tempered and angry—unreasonable response to things and people which would not usually bother the patient.
- Unrealistic demands and desires—a go-for-broke, devil-may-care attitude about material or financial matters or a to-hell-with-the consequences attitude toward physical matters.
- Hallucinations—imagining people, voices, and incidents, receiving nonexistent messages or hearing what is said incorrectly.
- The inability to grasp the meanings of messages or actions being said or done to him/her.
- A vagueness in a usually acute, alert mind.
- Lying about symptoms of pain and other physical manifestations.
- Answering questions according to what he/she feels is most acceptable to care-givers.
- Fear of expressing real feelings to care-givers and/or family.
- Lack of response to important issues and actions.
- Any aberrations of personality which may pass unnoticed by others who did not know the patient in a healthy state.

Many patients and their families are afraid, embarrassed or unable to admit and/or communicate their reactions and the effects of medication. Many accept weird symptoms as normal or feel that telling a doctor he or she is responding adversely to drugs or medication somehow insults the doctor or will be translated by care-givers as an unnecessary complaint or an indication of lack of faith. Each human being responds individually to drugs and medication. That is one reason there are so many varieties of drugs on the market today. Doctors and pharmacists want to cooperate with the patient and his/her family to find exactly which available drugs work best *if they know how the patient is responding.* It is up to you and the person who is ill to be aware of every abnormal drug response and report it immediately.

Remember, your observations and input are invaluable tools for your doctor and others caring for your loved one. One way to point out changes and receive the attention you feel may be needed is to stop at the nursing station, ask for the head nurse, and say, "I want it to be noted on this patient's chart and record that this is happening and is unusual for him or her. I shall expect the doctor to let me know what causes the problem and what is going to be done about it." Wait at the desk until the nurse has recorded your message, then wait eight hours and follow up on your notification to find out what has been done. Your ability to be assertive is important now and will become more important as time goes on.

It may be that you and your patient will have to accept odd behavior and hallucinations (as well as abusive language and actions you never dreamed of) as a consequence of allowing him/her to be pain-free through drugs. Many people have had to bear wrongful recriminations, false accusations, recitals of long-forgotten injuries and slights as well as unbelievably childish tantrums from a sick person on drugs. Often these changes and outbursts are so bizarre you cannot believe what is happening. Don't believe your ears! Do *not* believe your beloved person really *means* what he or she is saying. Know instead that this is the ranting of a bad dream in which she or he is caught. It is the drug or disease talking— not the person.

If you are hurting, don't strike back. Leave the room. Don't defend yourself. Simply tell your loved one, "I love you.

I'll come back in a little while," and *leave the room*. Don't waste energy and emotion in trying to reason with a nightmare. Bless them, forgive them and forget what they have said. An open wound will get infected and the entire process of healing will be prolonged.

If you leave *each time* you are confronted with a barrage of abuse, it will become evident that you will neither retaliate nor accept abuse, and you'll find nine times out of ten the tirades will cease. This change in your attitude and reaction toward the changes in your patient is difficult but necessary if you are to remain strong, useful and loving during trying times. This treatment for change of attitude has been tested and it works.

One phenomenon in terminal illness that can cause hurt and misunderstanding is the seeming *withdrawal* of the patient from loved ones. There appears to be a touch-me-not attitude or an invisible wall that cannot or will not be discussed by the ill person. This withdrawing is often misinterpreted as rejection.

Realize that withdrawal is a form of introspection and/or pre-death grieving. Accept the fact that a person who is terminally ill *must* go through this period in order to find the answers to his or her conditions of mind, body and spirit, and you will find that after withdrawal passes, he/she will be better able to cope with the everyday process of living until the end.

It seems cruel and mysterious that a loved one would withdraw from you when your time together is most precious, but think of it as a period when he or she is packing for a journey and needs time to gather up the loose ends of life. Your understanding, assurance, and constancy will make it easier for him or her to pass through this phase of illness. Your misunderstanding of this withdrawal will add to the guilts and frustrations of the process and can ultimately prolong the distance between you. Be patient. Accept.

While withdrawal causes hurt and misunderstandings, *indifference* is undoubtedly the most exasperating change of all. It can drive you up a wall when a person who has always had an opinion or preference mumbles, "I don't care" or "Do whatever you want to" or, worst of all, "It makes no difference to me, I'll not be around." At first, you are stunned by the apathy, then you are saddened, but finally you begin to suspect you are being victimized.

People who care for the terminally ill say indifferent responses can be an indication of depression, a power play, anger, fear, hostility, pouting, manipulation, rebellion or rejection. Whatever the reasons, the result is that you begin to resent their lack of interest in making decisions that should be jointly made. You resent being thrown the reins of power through default rather than appreciation and you are probably frightened by being thrust, ill-prepared, into a decision-making role.

Everyone who is ill needs to feel he or she still has control of things in his/her life and including them in the decision-making process enhances their psychological outlook despite their professed indifference. Diplomatic firmness can often break through this resistance. These methods of encouraging a patient to take action in decision-making without embarrassing confrontation have been proven valid:

1. In your own words say, "Unless you have a better idea on how to handle _____, I am going to _____."

2. "These are our possible choices as I see them: a. _____, b. _____, c. _____. Let me know which your prefer."

3. "Here is a short checklist of legal things we should have updated and recorded. Please tell me which you'd like to tackle first and we can take care of them one at a time."

4. "Your illness has made me realize how slipshod we've been about wills and property, etc. I'm having a will drawn up (or property transfer, etc.) for each of us."

Sometimes the terminally ill patient will resist making decisions despite reassurances from care-givers who say that patients feel better when they have resolved their problems and are "leaving their houses in order." To some patients signing a will or dictating a Letter of Intent indicates a resignation to their fate. Understanding their emotional needs is indeed important but survivors also need to have temporal matters clarified so that they can be relieved of unnecessary fears and frustrations now and later.

If you have reached a point where important joint and personal decisions *must* be made and the patient resists or withdraws, it is a kindness to yourself, your family and the patient to bring in a third respected party with the perspective and legal knowledge to explain the ramifications of legal documentation.

Your role as primary decision-maker may have already caused great stress and discomfort, and taking the helm of family finances during this emotional crisis can be downright frightening if it's new to you. But don't neglect those responsibilities! You cannot afford the complications of unpaid bills, ignorance of assets and liabilities, mortgages and obligations. Getting the information and instructions you need as soon as possible should be a Number One priority.

If you have never used a checking account or credit card, if you have no idea how bank statements are balanced or savings accounts are handled, go to your bank (savings and loan, credit union, broker, etc.). Ask to speak to the manager. He will find someone to provide the personal instructions you need to feel comfortable handling family finances. If you are a woman without a credit card or line of credit in *your* name ask that you be given a card at this time. Keep your spending to a minimum and ask for help if you have trouble understanding what you should do, how to do it or why it's important. (See page 105 on handling household finances and appointments.)

There are many men who for various reasons turn over the entire responsibility for family and household finances to their wives. When this person is faced with the dilemma of domestic expenses, he can generally get a clear idea of how the budget is set up by studying the family checkbook for the past three months. This method will usually tell which credit cards are being used, which charge accounts are active, where certain items are usually purchased, etc., and when payments are due.

Sometimes it is the better part of wisdom to ask a family

35

member or close friend to help out during the first few weeks when you take over the running of family finances. If someone will organize the bills, fill out checks for you to sign and mail them in on time, and balance your account, you will be spared one time-consuming job you do not need. If you have a friend who understands insurance policies and who will put those complicated forms and statements in order for tax purposes, you will have relieved yourself of one of the biggest financial headaches you will have to face.

Few husband/fathers are familiar with *all* the details of running a household. Child care, curricular routines, medical/dental appointments and other typically domestic matters seem to fall to a wife and mother even though she may be a working woman with an equally busy career.

Nevertheless, regardless of how well the surviving spouse (either husband or wife) may cook, do the laundry and take care of children's needs, there will be some things they simply should not attempt to do just now. This is why it is important to get a plan for home and child care in place as soon as possible. When the domestic scene is tranquil a family is better able to work on the larger problems which are certain to come along.

Children sense the stress and sorrow adults feel. Those who are overly protected from the gravity of the illness or who have been promised that "Mommy (or Daddy) will soon be all better" will surely lose confidence in adults when that promise cannot be kept. People who lower their voices or whisper in the presence of children build fear in the children. Children who are overly indulged, whose routines are interrupted, who find themselves being petted and pampered because of the illness of a family member may use pity as a manipulative tool long after the illness has been resolved. Children who are sent away, even for their own good, feel abandoned. Homes and familiar surroundings spell security. To be thrust into an alien household or to be isolated from everything and everyone a child holds dear could lead to residual complications.

Problems like these and the need for security should be carefully considered before children are removed from their homes or placed in a "protected environment." Children should take part in the decision-making process when it comes to their situation during a loved one's terminal illness. The psychological impact on them and the possible effects on their emotional life are far more important than the immediate convenience of surrounding adults.

A child who can snuggle down each night in a familiar bed, who is surrounded by the sounds and smells and shapes he or she loves is far less likely to have nightmares, wet the bed, or develop nervous twitches and antisocial behavioral problems.

Difficult as it may seem, it is far better for the surviving spouse to remain as independent as possible in a family crisis. It is wise to seek support but at the same time remain in charge of the household. Usually there is one close friend or family member who is familiar with the routines and tastes of the family—if that person will supervise hired help, many domestic problems can be avoided. This is a financial drain to be sure, but with the help of a Social Service agency, organized support groups, and health care agencies, domestic help can be found which can be trusted, and is usually competent and affordable.

Don't expect everything to be the same; your housekeeper may not do windows or shop with the care and acumen you're accustomed to. Often these extra jobs can be done by those loving people who ask: "What can I do to help?" Keep a list. Let them mend or babysit or bake a cake or give a birthday party or take the little one to the doctor, playground or circus. Friends like these will keep your family independent and if not happy, at least more confident and comfortable during this trial.

And speaking of lists, *be certain* to allow your spouse to cooperate in writing the things an employee should know about your home and children. The household will run more smoothly if the person taking care of Mark or Mary knows they get hyper on sweets, get hives from fish, should not be bathed more than three times a week because of dry skin, need a nightlight, won't eat peas, etc. When your housekeeper knows that groceries have been bought by bulk and stored in the back of the garage or that you share a freezer with a neighbor or any of the little idiosyncrasies you have, life will be that much smoother for all.

Take advantage of the wisdom that social service workers can offer you. They have the education and know-how as well as hands-on experience to guide you through this time when your perspective is out of kilter and theirs is in top form. Expect to make some mistakes. Correct them and move on.

A person torn by job requirements, the grave illness of a spouse and the care of home and children cannot indulge in the luxury of pride, self-pity or frustrations. The responsibilities are going to look insurmountable but they are not. If you are trying to bring order into the chaos of a home where your spouse and co-parent of your children is incurably ill, you will find these three suggestions helpful once you have sorted out your values and priorities:

1. Draw up a careful but flexible plan which includes the physical, emotional and financial needs of your family.
2. Know your assets and liabilities and locate sources of help before there is an emergency need—know your options.
3. Accept help from family, friends and society but maintain as much self-reliance as possible.

These are tough times and they demand strength and discipline. You will be tempted by self-pity and dependency but meet the challenges with courage and determination, and you will come through this hell with a sense of pride and worthiness that will be a lasting tribute to your loved ones, your courage and your love of family.

After a long period of illness, you may begin to notice that the sick room, the bed and the body have become the most important things in the world to a person who is terminally ill. It comes as a shock to realize that an outgoing vibrant person can become so totally absorbed by the limits of bodily functions and care. His or her needs, comfort and desires become the center of his/her universe and you find yourself on the outside looking in. When this happens, it will help to remember that the body, bed and room comprise the world's most important battleground right now for your loved one. What is happening beyond the confines of this illness is incidental to the enormity of the time and place in which he/she now lives.

It's not uncommon to hear someone say they traveled great distances at great expense and inconvenience to see a dying loved one only to be casually greeted and/or ignored. Others have said they were asked to leave so that the patient could sleep or watch a soap opera undisturbed. There is little etiquette when one is dying. Preoccupation with self and self-needs and desires is as natural to a terminally ill person as it is to a newborn infant.

There is a theory among those who care for the terminally ill that the less interested a patient becomes in the world beyond the sickbed, the easier it is to leave life. If that theory is correct, is it not foolish and self-defeating to allow ourselves to be hurt by or resentful of this natural leave-taking process? Life became much simpler for me when I learned I could best accept changes by altering my attitude and reaction to them. I found that by asking myself, "Can I do anything about this situation to change it?" If the answer was no, I made myself accept and/or dismiss it. If the answer was maybe, I'd spend some time thinking over possible answers and alternatives. If the answer was yes, I'd give the problem my full attention until I reached an acceptable solution.

Let's try my formula on one of the most common and disruptive problems we face when we know a loved one is dying. Doctors, for example, frequently give orders to a patient forbidding salt, smoking, fats, caffeine, sugar, and the like. Common sense tells us this advice is meritorious and the orders should be obeyed. While we may agree that doctor knows best, we know jolly well our mate or parent is not going to even consider doctor's orders, let alone obey them. We listen and watch him/her give lip service but we'd bet our bottom dollar that within twenty-four hours, orders will be ignored, belittled or ridiculed. The theory is great but the practice is not for our beloved.

How do we handle this everyday situation? What do we

say when a terminally ill patient argues, "I'm going to die anyway, why should I give up the few remaining pleasures of life?" We have to choose our answers carefully.

My introduction to the dilemma was Bob's smoking habit. My neighbor's problem was diet control for one she loved and another friend found forbidden bottles of vodka stashed in strange places. The three of us have faced the ordeal of watching someone we love deliberately and with forethought choose to shorten life rather than remain with us just a little longer.

I nagged, begged and policed. Bob made promises and broke them. I ranted and raved. His sons tried to convince him—all to no avail. It became an awful battle of wills. Even though he wouldn't smoke around me, I could smell cigarettes and knew he was sneaking smokes in the bathroom or out behind the house. It was a no-win battle until I realized that I couldn't change Bob. *We can only change ourselves.* I could either make these last few months miserable and guilt-ridden or I could accept this man's right to conduct his life and his habits as he saw fit. Indeed, as he kept insisting, it was his life.

I stopped nagging and brought out ashtrays. He continued smoking. We didn't discuss my surrender or his victory. When he'd light a cigarette and have a coughing fit, he'd grin and say, "It's those damned cigarettes" and I'd say, "Yup" and that was that. I don't know if the compromise on my part was right or wrong. Perhaps it hastened his death. I do know, however, that by acknowledging his rights and by choosing harmony over dissension, the last of our days together became a close, caring time I will always cherish.

Once you have made up your mind that you are not responsible for the negative behavior of others, you will find new freedom. You will discover the truth of the sages: One cannot live another's life nor die another's death.

There will be social and interpersonal changes during a terminal illness. You will soon differentiate between friends and acquaintances and what you can expect from each. It's your expectations that cause confusion—and sometimes bitterness—in relationships during this time of stress. If you can allow friends to separate themselves from acquaintances naturally, like cream rising to the top of milk, you will spare yourself the grief and disappointment that so often accompanies this period.

Friends are rare and beautiful—they will be with you in body, mind and spirit from the first diagnosis to the final sad parting. Acquaintances, on the other hand, are people who care but don't know what to do to be helpful during your time of need. Acquaintances relate serious illness and death to *other* people, not to themselves. The thought of death is discomforting and is to be avoided. Facing the reality of someone else's death forces them to face their own mortality. This is an irrational response and it hurts to be avoided by someone you thought a friend, but it is not an uncommon occurrence.

Life is simpler when we realize friends and acquaintances are like flowers—they come in annual and perennial varieties. Both add color and dimension to our lives and each fulfills specific needs at specific times. When we learn to accept and appreciate what each person can offer, not allowing our expectations or disappointment to clutter our lives, we find the bountiful rewards an unfettered relationship can bring.

One of the saddest phenomenon of a terminal illness is the discovery that some friends have become acquaintances. Deep, close friendships of many years can become strained and/or distant for no apparent reason. In the midst of your turmoil you will wonder what happened to a once cherished relationship—did he or she find you lacking? Did you offend? Where did you err? It is so easy to be oversensitive! It is tempting to accept the blame for any flaw in life. Don't allow yourself to accept guilt or to become the culprit of imagined difficulties. Accept the changed relationship without judgment if you can. The reason will become clear later when you've gained your equilibrium and perspective. Remember that true friends always reappear.

A friend of many years came to me after Bob's death and said, "I wanted so much to help you but I didn't want to intrude. I hurt for you but I could see you were managing well without me. You were so busy and tired, I didn't want to get in your way." I wish I had known she felt that way. I had missed her. I should have asked for her help because I know it would have meant a great deal for her to have felt useful and sharing. As it was, I shut her away from me by not considering *her* needs. We both lost through our blindness to each other's needs.

It takes a special kind of courage to ask for and offer help in difficult times, but it's in giving and receiving that real friendships are cemented. There are times when all of us have avoided helping someone we knew could use our help. Sometimes I find myself sending a note, card or flowers in lieu of a hospital visit simply because of the sad memories it evokes. Hospitals drain me emotionally and I avoid them to my embarrassment and shame.

We should be gentle in our judgments of others during difficult times, for ultimately *we* may be in need of gentle understanding from another. If a friend offers to step in to relieve you for an hour or a day, accept this relief quickly and with gratitude. You need time off during the prolonged illness of a loved one.

Often a new face around the care arena will stimulate the bed- or housebound. You both will benefit from this change. Too often we find ourselves playing hostess in a hospital or home-care setting. We forget the need to share and even to relinquish some of the care of a loved one to friends who may also need to help.

When friends ask, "How can I help you?" you may be caught off guard or in the difficult position of wanting to share but not wanting to overburden your relationship. One way of solving the problem is by keeping a list of chores you find easy to delegate (pick up dry cleaning, buy stamps, water plants, walk dog, contact people and/or organizations, etc.). Let them choose which jobs they'd like and you'll find their help fulfills mutual needs. Sharing chores and problems builds friendship when it is done with love and consideration.

If we shut out friends and acquaintances we isolate ourselves from a source of strength, which is necessary for our own endurance. There is truth in the proverb: "Friendships multiply joys and divide griefs."

CHAPTER·4

Stress

Stress is a fact of life. A certain amount of stress is even healthy. But the stress you are experiencing right now is frightening—it's unique to this terminal illness in which you're involved. This kind of stress will grow and devour you unless you acknowledge and deal with it as it happens, with both intelligence and with determination.

Your stress shows up in stiff muscles and neck and back pain. Stress is why your sleep is disturbed. It's why you find it difficult to concentrate. It's why you lose your car keys and your temper. Stress is why you can't remember names or telephone numbers or where the insurance policies are kept and why you don't give a damn about most things you once felt were important, such as your appearance, your work, your relationships both casual and close, your finances, your diet, your attitudes. At the time you need most to be in control, stress keeps you off base and feeling unnatural. And no wonder! This is a very unnatural time in your life. Never before have so many of your resources been called upon. You are being mentally, spiritually, financially, physically and emotionally stressed.

Unfortunately, it is not possible to remove the causes for your stress. It *is* possible and necessary to make them bearable and controllable. The secret is to realize what you can and cannot do about the various stresses you are facing.

Begin by acknowledging you *are* experiencing stress. Second, decide that you are going to handle the symptoms of stress with intelligence and determination *as they appear.*

Stoicism—really only hiding your stress from yourself—will only make you a slave to it.

Take note! You are in stress if:

- you have a desire to eat, drink or smoke more than you normally do.
- you experience a deep fatigue or malaise that sleep or rest doesn't alleviate.
- there is a knot in your stomach, a tightness in your chest, your teeth are clenched or you have a twitch in the corner of your eye or mouth.
- you find your hands are clenched or restless.
- you have trouble breathing or there is a dull ache in your solar plexus or near your heart.
- you have bad dreams or recurring nightmares.
- you sweat profusely or have chills.
- there are flu-like symptoms in muscles and joints.
- you have hives, itchy skin or a rash.
- you feel queasy—a kind of morning sickness that follows you through the day.
- you have diarrhea or unusual constipation.
- you crave certain kinds of foods.
- you become accident-prone.
- you are extremely sleepy or unnaturally hyperactive.
- you are abnormally forgetful or lacking in concentration.
- you experience deep fears of things that never frightened you before.
- you have the urge to run away or withdraw from people you normally like to be around.
- you are angry or let things bother you that never troubled you before.
- you have a deep, morbid unrelenting depression you cannot shake.
- you've lost your sense of humor and/or perspective.
- panic strikes and your heart pounds for little or no apparent reason.

These are but a *few* manifestations of stress!

If these symptoms are disrupting your life, or frightening you or your family, talk the situation over with your doctor. Accept his or her prescription and advice just as you would accept a brace if you had sprained your ankle. After that, help yourself to ease your stress so that you will not become too dependent on drugs or become habitually stressed.

Having faced great stress over a long period, I truly believe the "Prayer for Serenity" is one of the best stress-fighting tools there is. This prayer has a sound psychological basis and it may help if you contemplate its wisdom.

God grant me the serenity
To accept the things I cannot change
Courage to change the things I can
And the wisdom to know the difference.
                                        —Anon.

Ways You Can Relieve Stress

1. Take a short brisk walk, regardless of the weather. It need not be more than a ten-minute jaunt in the fresh air. Breathe deeply and swing your arms.

2. Soak in a warm tub, into which you have lavished your favorite fragrance, or dump in one-half cup of baking soda, which has a soothing effect. Lean back and allow yourself to float in mind and spirit. Think of only good things. If you start to cry, let it happen and then go back to your good and happy thoughts. If you begin to feel fearful, dismiss your fears and replace them with happier thoughts. Consider this quiet time in your bath as a gift from you to you. Breathe deeply and relax each muscle. By the time the tub is cool, you will be better able to face the world.

3. This stress reliever is a little tricky to explain but it works best of all! Sit *quietly* and allow yourself to think of all the blessings you still experience. Forget for a little while all the negative things

and be grateful for all the positive things surrounding you. Force yourself to be grateful for the small as well as the greatest blessings in your life for just a few minutes each day. If you do, you will emerge from this period refreshed and recharged.

4. Most anyone in the scientific community will tell you that stress is a basic cause of illness, or at least plays a major role in physical and mental problems. Because of that fact, it is *very important* to keep your body well nourished. The daily vitamin supplements I used and my decision to stay healthy carried me through the grueling months and years of stress I endured. I cut down on coffee, carbohydrates and empty calories and concentrated on food that would nourish me and rest lightly in a stomach that felt like I had swallowed a brick.

There is supporting evidence for giving your body the best care by way of good food, ample rest, exercise and supplemental vitamins. A candy bar, a peanut butter sandwich or doughnut and coffee may be expedient and may fill your stomach, but these kinds of things will ultimately catch up with you when you are under stress and at a time when you most need to be healthy and on top of things. Good food is as available as poor, empty-calorie food, even in hospital or clinic vending machines. Look for apples, oranges, milk, nuts, or crackers and cheese. If simple good food is unavailable, try to carry protein tablets and/or trail mix to munch when you get the hungries.

If solid food is impossible to swallow, a milkshake, egg nog, or a cup of soup will go down easily. Stress and caffeine are *not* good companions—one feeds upon the other until you are tight as a fiddle string. Control your caffeine and refined sugar consumption and you will find

you can relax better. Omit them completely if
you can.

5. Once or twice a week do something to change
your routine of hospital visits or care-giving—you
need to remove yourself from the grind. It's not
so difficult to get away if you plan ahead. There
will be people who regularly visit the ill person.
Make arrangements with them to visit so that
you can escape for a few hours. This will fulfill a
threefold need. First, it gives your patient and
visitors privacy and a sense of sharing; second, it
keeps the patient from feeling like a burden to
you; third, it gives you necessary time alone. It's
a kindness to allow friends to help you this way
and it really will give you the perspective you
need.

Use the time to really escape. Take a walk.
Go to chapel. Have an unhurried lunch or dinner
at a nice place with a friend who will buoy you
up. Get a facial or massage or have your hair
done. Shop, browse or take a nap. Play golf or
tennis or bowl. Do something leisurely. Whatever
it is, make sure it is something *you* want to do. At
first you might feel guilty and a little
uncomfortable but with practice you'll see the
wisdom in recreation during this time.

Giving you time is the kindest gift a friend
can give and, believe me, it is a salvation from
stress.

6. With your head and heart in turmoil, you will
forget and misplace so many things that you will
often feel as if you are losing your mind. Rest
assured, you are not! One way to sort out the
confusion is to keep a small notebook in which
you can jot down things you must remember as
they occur, such as items your patient needs to
bring from home, telephone calls you are
expected to make, bills that must be paid,
appointments that must be kept, letters that

should be written, problems that must be solved. I called this list my "Must Do List." If these things are written down, they can be crossed off as they are accomplished and you will feel more competent and in control of your life. As for keys and glasses, I was always misplacing them until I had duplicate keys made, which I left with a friend, and began to wear my glasses on an elastic band, which can be purchased in most drug stores. I put letters and bills in a big basket the minute I opened and read them so I knew where they were when I needed them on Monday morning—the irrevocable time I set aside for business matters.

7. If ever it was true that the show must go on, it's when you are the only one in charge! So on Monday (choose the best day for you) I *always* set aside an hour or two to do bookwork and answer letters. This was the time I paid bills if they were due, wrote those Thank You notes that had accumulated and did important telephoning. There was satisfaction for me in starting the week off with a clean slate. It gave me a modicum of comfort and removed the guilt of owing letters of appreciation to people who had been kind to us. If there were appointments to make, Monday was the day I made them. This was also the day I did the laundry and got my wardrobe in shape for the week. All this took only three or four hours and made me feel more in control of my life. This control was very important to me at a time when I had no control over what was happening elsewhere. It's the only way I could have worked full-time, freelanced and taken care of Bob and our home.

8. Perhaps the best way to relieve stress involves sharing with one friend all your frustrations and heartaches. The right friend will listen *with* understanding and *without* judgment, acting as a

48

sounding board for all your fears and trials. This
is one of the world's great stress removers.
If you haven't a friend or family member who can
fill this need, find a chaplain, minister, priest or
psychologist and unburden yourself to them.
They are sworn to keep your secrets if you tell
them it's "privileged information." Besides,
believe it or not, they've heard it all before. There
are times when you don't need advice but the
comfort of relieving yourself of the frustration. It
makes good sense to seek advice from experts and
comfort from a listener.

Choose your listener carefully, tell him/her
that you just want to unload and spare the rest
of the world the retelling of your concerns. I
bless the person I chose. She listened, forebore
telling me I was an utter ass, and gave me
comfort by letting me know she loved me and
was *absolutely positive* that I would be okay
and that she understood what I was saying.
She knew that this unloading was for me what
tears and temper tantrums are to other people.
To this day she has never reminded me of the
terrible stuff I spilled into her loving lap. Friends
on whom we can dump are a rarity. Many people
are so steeped in bits and pieces of pop psychol-
ogy and so quick to judge that when you find
someone who cares enough to simply listen,
nodding when and where necessary as you rant,
rave and give vent to sorrow, you must cherish
and keep him or her. These folk are worth their
weight in gold.

If you don't have a friend who can listen and
forget, try writing your frustrations down. Study
and analyze them. You will find release and often
the perspective you need to handle them with
poise and composure. Then burn the paper—it
will have served its purpose. Often just getting
your resentments down on paper and out of your

system is all that's needed to help you see that most of them can be handled.

9. Take the above suggestion one step further if you still need help. Enumerate your problems on one half of a sheet of paper. Then on the other half list what you can do to remedy the situation. Try it on a simple scale. For instance, say the problem is that you are angry because you feel the doctors aren't being honest with you. Remedy: (a) You can go to them and tell them you resent their attitude. (b) You can ask to have another doctor put on the case and tell him/her you want and need a forthright opinion. (c) You can allow the problem to fester. (d) You can do some research in the library on your own. (e) You can question other care-givers (nurses, resident physicians, etc.). (f) Any other options you can think of.

When this is done, you will have a clearer picture of not only the problems but possible solutions. Follow through on the decisions you make and the burden of stress becomes lighter. The problem-and-solution method was a godsend to me. I felt so alone when I came back from visiting at the hospital or when there was a conflict between Bob and me over what was happening to him, me and us. Or if I was angry at the doctor or God (not necessarily in that order). Seeing on paper what was *really* troubling me allowed me choices. Focusing on my options allowed me to solve the problem in a way best suited to my needs.

10. The last good advice is probably the most difficult: the practical decisions that must be met and acted upon. You are going to have to know certain pragmatic things and solve practical problems. If you and your mate have never had a will drawn up or do not know about family insurance policies, bank accounts, stocks or bonds

and/or other investments which will have to be dealt with, now is the time to do it. We'll cover the details later in the chapter on "Very Important Papers," but it cannot be emphasized strongly enough that knowing your whole financial story in advance will save a great deal of heart and headache later on.

Difficult as it may be, talk to an attorney and find out what steps should be taken *immediately* as to updating or writing a will for *both of you* if you are husband and wife, or if the person who is ill is a parent. Check into Power of Attorney, Survivor Clauses on property, pension or stock plans which may be involved in employment, insurance policies, etc. Your lawyer will know what should be done.

I found that by working out the financial puzzle in such a way as if *I* were dying, it was far easier for me to approach the subject of wills to Bob. It's terribly difficult to discuss death and wills with a terminally ill loved one but it's also terribly important. Once you have resolved these practical questions, you will feel more relaxed. While you are on the subject of wills and Powers of Attorney, it is a good time to find out if *both* of you opt to donate to an organ bank.

This is also the time to decide on The Living Will (a copy will be found in the back of the book). If you and the patient are not willing to have life sustained by artificial means, you must let it be known. Put your wishes *on record*. If you feel strongly that *quality* of life is more important than the prolongation of it, be *sure* that the doctor and hospital know. Put a record of your wishes in the hands of the care-givers and family members. If these difficult decisions are made ahead of time, you will be saved further stress and turmoil later, for you will have *proof* that you are doing what your loved one requested

51

when he/she was lucid and able to make decisions.

People who have gone through the ordeal of a terminal illness often say that just when they believed they had reached the limit of their endurance, someone or something came into their life and brought them new strength and faith. Had it not happened to me, I might discount it as grasping at straws. Now, though, I'm inclined to think of these incidents as a special kind of miracle.

I badgered God until He must have been tired of the harangue. I had come to the conclusion that if there was a God, He, She or It was either beyond reach or didn't give a damn. I would not "trouble deaf heaven with my bootless cries." Bob's coming death was certain and slow and we were both tired of the whole process. It was one of those rare and beautiful clear blue days of February and I needed to escape from my world. I called the dog and we went for a walk. I had never walked along the railroad, and so, for a change of scenery we headed up the tracks. Katrina bounded along ahead of me and a puff of wind blew a piece of paper off a wild rose bush and tumbled it along the gravel bed. Kat pounced on it and brought it back to me to toss so that she could retrieve it.

I'm the sort of person who *must* read anything printed. It was a weathered page from a pulp magazine about the size of *Reader's Digest*. Winter had obliterated all but a corner, which read "as a child: Trust in the Lord with all thine heart and rely not on thine own understanding. Acknowledge him in all ways and he will direct thy path." Obviously it was a passage from the Bible, so I tore it off and stuck it in my pocket, intending to see if I could find its place when I got home. I threw the remainder for the dog· and continued the walk, forgetting all about it until I turned the pockets of my jacket on wash day. I looked in Proverbs and Psalms because they seemed the logical places for such a passage, but the search was time-consuming and I left the torn corner in the Bible and got busy with other things.

Spring came. On Mothers' Day my eldest son and his family came to visit me. My grandchildren and I have a favorite rock overlooking the river, and while we were sitting on that rock, taking turns singing favorite songs they startled me by singing "Trust in the Lord with all thine heart . . ." "Where did you learn that?" I asked. "Where does it come from?" "I don't know," they answered, "but Daddy will know." When we went home we asked and Bill gave me chapter and verse and sure enough! There it was. So I left the tattered corner between the pages and went back to my busy world.

Bob and I had decided if it was at all possible we would go home to New England for one last visit with family and friends. Since there was to be a wedding and the whole clan would be together, we made arrangements for oxygen and wheelchairs and the other paraphernalia it would take to get there and stay for a short visit. We flew to Boston and after a few days, Bob took a turn for the worse and had to be hospitalized. I was frantic, but the doctors and nurses were wonderful and the family was supportive and kind beyond belief.

It was a muggy afternoon as I sat beside the bed in Exeter. Bob was sleeping and I decided to walk about town for a few minutes. On my walk I passed a bookstore and went in to browse, hoping to find something effortless to read. A woman asked if she could help me and I declined. I didn't find anything and started to leave when she came up to me. She smiled and said, "Excuse me, I don't mean to intrude my dear, but you do look so tired." I explained that I was from Oregon and my husband was hospitalized. She said she was sorry and *then* she said, "You know, I'm not a religious person in the strictest sense but I've had a few bad times in my life and there is a proverb that has helped me over the humps of life. 'Trust in the Lord with all thine heart and rely not on thine own understanding. Acknowledge him in all ways and He will direct thy path.' "

I laughed and gave her a big hug. I told her about finding that very same Proverb on the railroad tracks, hearing it sung by Jessica, Kristen and Seth and now, thousands of miles from Portland, here it was again! I tore back to the hospital convinced that it was a sign. Trust in the Lord (metaphysically

53

"Lord" means "law"). That proverb became imprinted on my mind and heart and carried me through to the bitter end of Bob's illness. It was the beginning of my acceptance and understanding that when there was nothing I could do, I must trust, and that there was direction and help. I'm not a Bible thumper, and I too could not be called a religious person in the narrow definition, but I firmly belief that whether you call it God's voice, coincidence, a talisman, or simply an answer, it was what I needed at the perfect time and place. A friend said he lived by the saying: "This, too, will pass." Another friend of mine said she got through her greatest period of stress on this bit of wisdom: "Yesterday is but a dream and tomorrow is only a vision but today was a real bitch. What am I going to do about it?"

If you look, you will find a comforting quotation, talisman or mantra that will relieve your stress and carry you through. The secret is looking and believing, and trying to handle stressful problems one at a time as they present themselves.

CHAPTER 5

Support Systems (Friends and Helpers)

To many people, the term "support system" sounds stuffy and inhibiting. The truth is, a support system could be one of your greatest blessings. A support system is a group of giving, caring, understanding, experienced and helpful people joined together in their dedication to help others through difficult times.

Support systems seldom intrude. They welcome you, offer assistance and a place to bring your problems—whether large or small. Once you are aware of what they offer, you may choose to join them or go it alone. In any case, it is comforting to know there are people out there who will listen, understand, and help.

The need for support systems became greater as families became more fragmented and mobile and as homes became smaller and less adaptive to nursing care. We can no longer depend on family, neighbors or a tight-knit community to rally 'round and support us in a time of need. We have fewer family doctors and clergy today, leaving us to go to strangers with our physical, spiritual and emotional problems. We must create our own "communities." Seek out available support systems *early* in a terminal illness so that when and if we need their strength, we can call on them immediately.

Spiritual help and support can be found through almost

all churches and synagogues nationwide. Some religious denominations and organizations have toll-free, twenty-four-hour counseling services, staffed with trained lay people to assist you in difficult periods. There are also small, intimate prayer circles within many local churches as well as prayer lines (telephone numbers) where Biblical and inspirational passages are recorded. Many churches have on-call clergy to help you on a round-the-clock basis. You can find the spiritual help you need simply by asking at any church or synagogue or by calling church offices listed in the Yellow Pages of your telephone directory.

Emotional crisis support groups ar also readily available. They can be located by calling your local Mental Health Service, Human Resources, Family Services, or the Social Services in the Yellow Pages. You need not go into detail when you contact these people. Simply say, "I am looking for help." They will quickly put you in contact with the proper agency.

Many hospitals, clinics, churches and synagogues offer their premises to support groups which have been formed to guide families of the terminally ill throughout the illness. Hospice organizations have done an outstanding job of guidance and counseling; the American Cancer Society, Red Cross, Visiting Nurses Association, Salvation Army Services and many more religious and nonprofit organizations such as those listed on pages 182 to 201 are willing not only to help you find guidance during this time, but can offer you understandable information about various treatments for the disease with which you are involved.

In almost every community there are small informal groups of people who have suffered or are suffering the loss of a loved one. In many instances these people, who know firsthand the stresses, crises, emotions and desperations you are experiencing, can be of far greater comfort and value than people who have not experienced them. Here is a place where you can vent your deepest concerns without fear of censor. Here you are made comfortable by the knowledge that everyone in the room completely understands your suffering. You are accepted at face value and allowed to *be* who you are without pressure; you can be as active or passive as you choose.

One man explained to me when I visited a hospice-sponsored support group, "We are the walking wounded and for the most part we're afraid to show how deeply we're hurt or how much we need comfort. Here, in this group, I've learned to say I'm scared, or guilty or just damn angry. Here I can openly admit without shame that I resent having my needs ignored while everyone focuses on the needs of my wife. Here we can explore ways of getting rid of negatives and find ways of changing destructive behavior into positive action. We help each other find better ways of communicating with our families and our loved ones. Each person here knows the terrible pain of watching someone we love die and we all know the frustration of not being able to postpone their departure.

"In my case it's my wife who is dying. Our kids are losing a mother and I'm losing a friend and a wife. We couldn't talk about it because we were hurting too badly. We came and listened to others talk about how they felt and what they did to make it better. It took a couple of weeks and then gradually we began listening to each other and discussing our feelings openly. It's been a godsend."

A woman who joined Candlelighters (a support group for families of children with cancer) said, "I was convinced I was cracking up! I'd forget things. I didn't hear what people said to me even as they spoke. I'd cry or laugh over nothing at all. I was wacko! I'd wake up shaking and sweating. I balked at joining any group, let alone one that would talk about what I couldn't even face. But my husband and a friend went with me and it wasn't long before I realized that everyone in that room had felt what I was feeling. I saw people as hurting as me who had actually survived! I saw people who turned from desperation to hope and mostly I saw the value of living each day at a time and making the most of it. I learned the value of *now* and I saw how this group celebrated life right now within the confines cancer had placed on them. It didn't take long for me to choose to make the most of the life we had. Now when I get scared or depressed I'm not ashamed to admit it and do something about it. And it's helped make us a team here at home. We can talk more openly about the problems of chemotherapy and we can go on picnics, hayrides and pizza parties with other parents and with kids who are facing bone marrow tests, loss of hair, sick stomachs and all the bad stuff without having to explain or hide our concerns. When anyone in the group needs support, we're there. When we need support, they're there. It really makes a difference."

Probably the most helpful support system is friends. In reading all the books I could find on personal crisis, stress, grief and how to cope with them, there was one need that came through loud and clear—the need for at least one supportive friend. That friend will be your anchor in the storm. He or she will be an unobtrusive lifesaver and perhaps even the key to your survival. How do you tell who is a supportive friend? Here is the distillation of dozens of books and definitions:

A supportive friend—

1. will be there when and as you need. Your calls will be welcomed and it will be easy to unload your burden of mental, emotional, psychological, and spiritual problems, knowing your friend will remain far enough removed from the problems to feed back to you the perspective you may have lost.
2. is not shocked or judgmental when you express depressing or negative thoughts and will accept your tears and your anger as natural human reactions to your situation.
3. is warm and affectionate but not maudlin, thus allowing you to use his/her strength as a support—not a pillow or sponge.
4. offers advice only when it is asked for and is not miffed when you disregard it, thus allowing you freedom of choice (knowing it is your confusion and not your lack of intelligence which causes you to choose the wrong things).
5. considers your needs and tries to provide for them quietly and without fanfare.

6. can easily communicate with other friends who want to be helpful without seeming to be overprotective or demanding.

7. will shield you from chores which another person can do but which may be draining or difficult for you.

8. will try to bring you as much happiness as possible. Maintains an upbeat attitude without being a Pollyanna.

9. respects your need for privacy but remains available.

10. believes in your ability to overcome adversity and trusts you to do your best.

Sometimes it's hard to remember that everyday chores that consume your time and energy can be easily handled by other people who would be grateful to show in a more tangible way that they care. It is a kindness on your part to let them help. Remember that friendships strengthen by thoughtful use. The time will come when you can reciprocate. When you are asked, "What can I do for you?" tell them! Thank them! Bless them! And always remember their kindnesses.

If you are not actively involved in the care of a terminally ill person, here are a few helpful suggestions that never fail to lighten the burden of the care-giver. Choose one or two and make them your job.

Pet Care:
Walk the dog, play fetch, brush or wash the dog (or take him/her to the groomer). If there is a litter box, change the litter. If the dog/cat/bird needs shots or veterinarian care, be the one to take it. Bird cages and aquariums are easy to clean— offer to do it. If the animal is suffering from loneliness or neglect, take it home with you.

Plant Care:
Water houseplants, mow the lawn, trim the bushes, sweep the walk, water the lawn and garden, fertilize if necessary. Rake leaves or shovel snow, depending on the season.

Home Care:
Vacuum, dust, change linens, do a few loads of laundry, fold towels and sheets, mend, sew on buttons, do special laundry tasks (bedjackets, nighties, p.j.'s, bed socks), empty the trash, wash windows, defrost the refrigerator, take dry cleaning out or pick it up, shop for groceries, pick up necessary prescriptions, cook a meal. Return casserole dishes to people who have sent food and thank them.

Car Care:
Take the car to a garage for lube job and/or oil change when needed. Wash and wax the car (just a run-through at a car wash helps). Vacuum and empty ash trays, clean windows, check tires, change and rotate tires in season. Offer to chauffeur your friend when and as needed.

Child Care:
Babysit or take a child or two into your home for a day or two *if they will be happy and comfortable.* Take children to the theater, zoo or park for an outing (they love to include one or two of their friends and it makes caring for them easier). Give a child small gifts that encourage quiet play—coloring books, puzzles, games, tapes, records, stickers and sticker books. Books the child can read or books you offer to read to them are always special. Wrap your gifts in happy paper with bright ribbons. Even the simplest gift becomes special. Let a child decide what he or she would like to do on a special outing. Go out to lunch or dinner with a child, but try to avoid sweets. Some kids get hyper from them. Most children love video games. You might rent an enchanting movie if the family has the proper equipment.

Gifts Other Than Flowers and Cards and Balloons:
- A gift certificate at a favorite deli or bakery.
- A cheesecake or torte that will keep in the refrigerator until needed.
- Theater tickets with a note promising to stay with the patient as long as needed.

- Reservations at a resort or hotel for a weekend of R and R for the care-giver.
- Gift certificates for a massage, facial, manicure or hairdo.
- Pleasant teas or coffees.
- Note paper or informal cards with stamps.
- Brandy or wine for that end-of-the-day sipping.
- Easy-to-read books.
- Care packages of easy-to-fix, nourishing foods.
- Home-made soups, baked goods, casseroles, etc. that can be frozen and eaten when needed.
- A roast, fried chicken, ham or cold cuts.
- Snacks in small packages that can be tucked into a pocket or purse for munching on the run.
- A special soap, bath salts, powder or lotion.
- A funny card or T-shirt.
- Placing your friends in a prayer circle or on a prayer list or special service according to their beliefs or yours—and letting them know they're in your prayers.
- Crossword puzzle magazines or word games if your friend likes them.
- A hug. Always give hugs. Everybody needs hugs when they're tired and worried.

Organize Groups of Helpers:
Organize friends, relatives and/or church members to provide meals and home services for a family who must spend a great deal of time at the hospital. Tape names on dishes or keep a list of meal descriptions so thank you notes will be appropriate. Set a designated time so that someone will be at home to accept your kindnesses.

Shopping and Errands:
Time and economy are two important factors to be considered during a terminal illness. If you can arrange to pick up the grocery list and shop once a week for the person who is homebound, it will be a great help. It's important to find out if a specific brand is preferable and to keep an accurate

account of the cost with proper change when you are reimbursed.

There are times when prescriptions will need to be changed or renewed, when new sickroom equipment needs to be purchased or other shopping done. If you volunteer to do these quick and easy chores, be sure that you have the proper receipts. Every item is tax-deductible and becomes more and more important as medical bills mount. *Save the receipts.*

Telephoning and Letter Writing:
There are always people who should be contacted during a terminal illness, but when under pressure, the primary caregiver has neither the time nor the emotional surplus to notify or update friends who care. Offer to call these people. Get explicit directions on how much or how little they are to be told of the condition. Be diplomatic if you are being pressured by the people you call. A vague reply such as, Really, I don't think a definite decision has been made" or "To be frank, I didn't feel I should ask about that just now" will usually indicate that privacy is desired.

There will be thank you notes and letters to be written. Offer to address and stamp envelopes if you feel unqualified to write them. There are forms you can follow to express the family's thanks and an informal sentence or two letting friends know that John or Mary is okay and will write when they can, really does wonders in keeping the guilts away.

Special Occasions:
When there is a terminal illness during special holidays or anniversaries, it is important that they be shared. To be sure, there will be a certain amount of wistful memories and there may be a lethargic response to celebrating during this difficult period, but sad as it is, to include and remember your friend will keep a deep, devastating loneliness and depression from overwhelming him/her.

Offer to Find Special Help if Necessary:
Sometimes it's easier for a friend to ask for assistance or to get advice or hire help than it is for people more emotionally

involved in the illness. If you know there are hospice and/or respite programs available and who to call, which rental agencies to contact for sickroom equipment, if there is a well-qualified pool of help on which to call, *you* are comforting the care-giver because *they* know you will have the proper information if and when it is needed. You will find that these humble offerings to find help can mean the difference between coping with the pressures of an illness or being swept under by them. Think of them as the widow's mite—the quiet gift of caring is always service.

Helpful support people will assist in the practical realities surrounding the time of death by providing information regarding wills, insurance policies, planning funerals, letters of intent and other arrangements in a way that is acceptable to both the family and the person who is dying.

Because of long experience with the psychological, emotional and physical changes that occur in the terminally ill as well as in the family, support groups can help everyone understand the various phases of impending death through group and one-on-one discussions. When the struggle is over support groups help families through the transitions of death. They know the organizations and people to call during the grieving or adjustment periods if they are needed.

Most support groups are non-profit or their fees are scaled to fit the individual's ability to pay. The United Way, Cancer Society, or Human Services Department in the hospital can easily put you in touch with an appropriate group. One tribute to these groups is that those who have availed themselves of their services have stated without exception that they intend to become a part of the programs which were so helpful to them.

PART·TWO

Options for Care

CHAPTER·6

Doctors, Communication, and Understanding

When Pope John died and went to heaven, he was met at the Pearly Gates by St. Peter, who showed him around the place.

Finally, after being taken to his quarters, St. Peter said, "Your Holiness, Heaven will be quite a change for you, but it's important for you to know that here in Heaven all things are equal. You see, in order to come here everyone was equally virtuous and so it stands to reason that everyone will be treated equally.

"There are no firsts or lasts here. We simply take turns, share equally, etc. Do you understand?"

"Oh, my goodness, yes!" exclaimed Pope John. "It's a wonderful idea, and to begin with you must call me John, not 'Pope' and not 'Holiness.' Right?"

"That's right. Any other questions? If not, I'll fly back to the Gate for our next arrival. Make yourself at home and I'll see you at lunch at the Celestial Cafeteria."

John spent a happy morning exploring Heaven, and when the Heavenly Chimes rang at noon, he joined a group of people waiting patiently to be served at the Celestial Cafeteria. All of a sudden, from around the corner comes a man in a white jacket who jumped in front of the first person in line. John noted the action and when St. Peter joined him, he said, "Didn't you say *everyone* was equal here?"

"Yes," answered St. Peter, *"everyone* is equal in Heaven. Why do you ask?"

"Well, I don't think the rule is working. For instance, I just saw a man come around the corner and place himself ahead of everyone in line."

"Was he wearing a white jacket?"

"Yes."

"Did he have a stethoscope in his pocket?"

"Come to think about it, he did have a stethoscope in his pocket."

"Oh," chuckled St. Peter, "don't let that bother you. That was God. He loves to play doctor."

When you feel intimidated by attending physicians, don't let it bother you. Remember that doctors like to play God!

Doctors, like all mortals, come in every size, shape, color, gender, specialty and skill. Finding the best doctor is, I believe, a matter of great luck and perseverance. If you have a doctor in whom you have perfect trust and rapport, cling to him! Cherish him! (This paragon may be a SHE of course.) Think of your doctor as a paid guide through the difficult journey ahead, for you will have to put your faith and the life of your loved one in his hands.

If you do not have a family physician to guide you, or if you are not satisfied with the attending physician, there are tried and true methods of finding the right doctor to take care of someone who is ill.

Many G.P.'s or family physicians will give you a referral list from which to choose a doctor. This may be satisfactory to the medical profession but it leaves much to be desired for the family and terminally ill patient, who want the most skilled, knowledgeable and compassionate professional in the business. They need someone they can trust, someone with empathy.

Before you zero in on any one doctor, check him/her out with professional health workers (nurses, other doctors, people who have had experience with him or her). This practical approach never occurs to people who would often give ten times the consideration to their mechanic or plumber than to the employment of a physician! A proven way to find someone

who is tops in his/her field is to make inquiries at universities or medical schools in your area. Many of the best doctors in private practice are affiliated with or teach in these institutions. You will usually find the latest medical procedures in these places.

Never accept the first diagnosis in a serious illness. Get a second opinion from another doctor (preferably a specialist) who is not affiliated with the clinic or hospital connected with the doctor who gave the first opinion—you will be assured of unbiased results. This is simply a good business practice and should not reflect your opinion of the doctors involved. In fact, most physicians welcome a second opinion and discussions of treatment options. Very few egos will suffer when you tell doctors you are seeking a second opinion.

It's a tall order for any doctor to meet the needs of both his patient and his patient's family but it can and should be done. After all, a practicing physician has chosen a profession that requires more than a technical approach to the problem.

While I realize there should be professional *perspective*, there IS a difference between perspective and detachment or indifference—and that is the area of greatest complaint among those of us who are dealing with the terminal illness. Each patient belongs to a family unit which is also suffering and whose emotional connections bring important responses from a patient. Any physician disassociating himself from the humanitarian needs of a patient is a technician, and should find an intermediary to communicate with his/her patient and the family.

If the patient will not readily admit to discomfort or pain, or is fearful, neurotic, hypersensitive, extremely modest, rigid in certain beliefs or has behavioral problems, handicaps, holds certain taboos or prejudices (even irrational ones), his/her doctor has the right to know them and it's your duty to tell him. If there is a deep fear of anesthetics, needles, difficulty in taking pills, allergies, dietary difficulties or preferences, a basic need for privacy or for companionship, all of these things should be spelled out from the beginning of your relationship with the person who will be taking care of the one you love.

69

In discussions with doctors and the families of dying patients, and from my own experience, I've found that the greatest discomfort and dissatisfaction on everyone's part in terminal illness is a lack of communication. Doctors say they have explained all the ramifications of the illness in detail, and families swear they were "never told." This disconnection in communication leads to all manner of misunderstandings.

Tell your physician what you expect from him and his colleagues. Make it clear and unmistakable that you expect honesty, compassion, and an understanding of the abstract needs of the patient and your family.

Facing reality is not simple at the onset of a terminal illness. Emotions are in a turmoil and fear is an ever-present companion. Because you need to know the *entire* scope of this illness, and because you are naturally in a state of confusion, it is important that there be someone to accompany you who can really listen to the doctor, who can understand what is being said and will remember the details. There will be questions you should ask or which should be asked for you. A friend or family member can ask them more comfortably than you can at this time. This backup system proves invaluable when you may be too stressed to absorb vital information. Because conferences with specialists are usually set for a specific time and place, a tape recorder used unobtrusively is quite acceptable to most physicians if they understand that you will need it for future reference. Simply say you're having problems remembering things just now and tape the meeting.

The greatest problem of communication is the illusion that it has been achieved. Communication is a key issue among patients, care-givers and physicians. If we cannot understand each other or what is going on, why not spend just a little time in clarifying what we want, what we mean and how we feel? Nothing is as fruitless as a conference in which nothing has any meaning. *Expect* to ask questions and be prepared by having them written down so that you can refer to them now and later. *Expect* your questions to be answered and not allow yourself to be deterred by fear of authority. Remember, *you* are *employing* these care-givers.

You have the *right* to question and they *owe* you the answers to your questions. Until you truly understand each other at this conference, communication has not been achieved.

These are the questions that should be asked by you and answered by the doctor from the beginning of any illness:

1. What *exactly* is the diagnosis?
2. What is the prognosis (future)?
3. What are the immediate consequences to be expected from the illness?
4. What will the treatment be?
5. What are the alternative treatments?
6. What will be the expected side effects?
7. Where does the physician believe is the best place for the patient to be treated?
8. Will the doctor accept and honor the Living Will or any special directives the patient and/or family have regarding treatments or life support preferences? Medical Power of Attorney and the Living Will should be photocopied and given at this time. (See pages 170 to 175.)
9. Are there important personality or psychological and physiological aspects in the patient which should be considered? (Phobias, philosophies, religious beliefs, fears, superstitions, allergies, etc.). Spell out these things to the doctor.
10. Express your feelings and explain your needs. (Any doctor treating the terminally ill should realize that the *people* as well as the disease must come into consideration.)
11. If after hospital treatment the patient will return home, what will (or should) the outpatient care be? If you will be caring for the patient at home, *insist* on clearly written directions over and above what is written on the prescriptions being used and *insist* on knowing all possible side effects of medication. *Insist* on knowing what you might logically expect to happen as the illness progresses. If there are any key symptoms of

which you should be aware, ask for a concise and understandable description of them. If you do not understand the medical terminology, for heaven's sake *ask questions!* It is amazing how many people really do not understand what a doctor is saying and are too embarrassed to ask. If a mechanic uses terms we don't understand, we don't hesitate to ask questions. Why then should we not question the physicians we have hired for the most important job of our lives? Medicine is a technical field, but the rudiments of its science can be explained in layman terms, if you *insist.*

12. If you have present or future financial needs, talk them out at this meeting. Doctors are prone to see only the treatment of the disease as their responsibility but they have at their disposal many names of people and organizations which can relieve families of unnecessary financial and emotional stress. A doctor can direct you to support systems, funding, low-cost (generic) prescriptions, free or minimum-cost equipment centers and many other helpful resources. Or your doctor can direct you to people who are familiar with these important resources. Unless you express the need, there is a tacit understanding among doctors and care-givers that you can resolve these problems yourself.

13. These are specific questions you should ask the doctor about medication suggested by Paul G. Rogers (National Council on Patient Information and Education):

(a) What is the name of the drug and what is it supposed to do?

(b) How and when should it be taken and for how long?

(c) What food, drink and other medicines or activities should be avoided while taking this drug?

(d) Are there side effects, and what should be done if they occur?

(e) Is there any written information available about this drug?

Keep in mind that doctors are *people*, just like you and me. Remember that they are in the business of healing disease and that failure to heal is hurtful to them. You and your family are but one unit of hundreds they must deal with and unless you enunciate your concerns, they cannot know them. Again I stress: *The greatest problem of communication is the illusion that it has been achieved. It is up to you to see that communication is achieved*, by asking questions, receiving answers, and understanding them.

Once you know and understand, you must face the dilemma of communicating the message to your loved ones. The decision to tell a terminally ill patient that this is a critical situation while still maintaining the necessary ingredient of hope is a delicate one and the debate over whether a person should be told about a terminal illness will probably go on forever. There are those who feel that knowing the truth of the gravity of the situation allows a patient to resolve conflicts, get affairs in order and make choices important to him or her. Dr. Kubler-Ross feels it is imperative that patients are told they are dying and I am inclined to agree.

How, by whom and when a patient is told about impending death are personal matters. It is astonishing how often I have been told that the patient brings up the subject casually or alludes to it in a roundabout manner, through a philosophic statement or by mentioning another patient who is facing death. My husband acknowledged his impending death by asking me to be sure his personal possessions were given to certain people. Others have said they were confronted by a patient asking to see an attorney, priest or special friend. There will be signals. If you listen carefully you will know when to talk of death with your loved one.

There are gentle ways of telling a patient he or she is facing death. Most hospitals have someone on the staff who is emotionally, spiritually and/or psychologically trained and able to meet the challenge. The doctor or nurses have probably attended seminars on death and dying, or have had enough

73

experience and tact to be able to discuss the situation with a patient in a logical and gentle way. And of course the clergy is trained in matters of dying, grief and communication. Who, when, and how to talk with a patient who is dying should be discussed early on with the doctor in charge when the prognosis has been given.

No matter how diplomatic or well prepared you think you are, no matter how brave, stoic, fatalistic, religious, or philosophic, when you realize that death is near, it is a soul-racking and heart-crushing time. You must gather all the resources you have collected over the years and face the truth. This is when family and closest friends can and should meld into a force that can enrich and sustain both you and your loved one until the final day. This is the reason clear communication with a doctor pays off, for it is the doctor who has the final control in the treatment of terminal illness.

CHAPTER · 7

Hospitals

The Business of Hospitals

Hospitals and hospital personnel are a world unto themselves. They are an industry, a business, and a bureaucracy. Some are non-profit, some are teaching facilities, and some are strictly profit-making concerns. They are indispensable. They are competitive. They are service-oriented. They are dedicated to compassion, religion, and/or science. Many are corporations, and yet most hospitals try to incorporate science, compassion, and healing into a humane but profitable organization.

The basic aim of all hospitals has been to heal the sick; only recently has the need to accommodate people facing a prolonged period of dying become an adjunct to hospital care. In the past the cost factor dictated that terminally ill patients be shuttled into nursing homes or convalescent facilities, but with more and more insurance companies and now Medicare accepting the costs of care for the terminally ill, many hospitals are including both in-patient and out-patient hospice care in their services. (See "Hospices.")

In dealing with hospitals over a period of time, it becomes necessary to understand the complex efficiency of its organization in order to utilize the services they offer. A *general* overview of hospital organization will help you find your way to services you may require. They are often organized as follows:

Boards of Trustees

Executives

(Development, Public Information, Community Education, Financial, Policy, Medical Records, Education, Human Resources, Department of Nursing, various specialized departments under Professional Support, and Business Departments which purchase and maintain the facilities)

Chiefs of Staff

Resident Staff Physicians

Affiliated Physicians

Affiliated Specialists

Head Nurse

Floor Nurses

Lab Technicians

Licensed Practical Nurses

Therapists

Nurses' Aides and Orderlies

Clerks

Maids and Cleaning Staff

Accountants

Chaplain and Chaplain Assistants

Volunteer Workers ("Grey Ladies," "Candy Stripers," etc.)

The people you will probably deal with will be your doctor and specialists, resident doctors, interns, head nurse, floor nurses, LPN's, aides, and possibly the chaplain, social workers, volunteer workers, plus, of course, the Accounting Department.

The very rich and very poor are usually assured of hospital coverage and it often surprises middle-income families to find that they, too, can be rescued from financial disaster for the asking. There has been legislation in most states written and acted upon to help defray the high cost of health care, and it is up to those of us caught in the bind of insur-

mountable hospital bills to ask for and receive the financial assistance we have paid for through taxes and voluntary donations.

State Human Resources Departments know of these available funds and can guide you through the steps it takes to get relief. If there is no Human Resources assistance in your area, call your county, state, or federal representatives, explain your situation to him or her, and ask for help. Don't let foolish pride of the moment deprive you of salvaging the property and savings of a lifetime. The Hill-Burton Act provides relief; see if you qualify. (See page 101, Hospital Costs—Hill-Burton Act.)

Conflicts with hospitals arise when we are not familiar with the services they offer or when they in turn are not aware of our needs. This state of affairs is rapidly and rightly changing as we make our needs known by communicating them through proper channels. Hospital competition forces the need for better customer relations. Many hospitals now have one person called the Patient Representative, whose duty it is to act as intermediary between patients (now called customers, consumers, or clients) and the care-givers. It is his/her function to see that patients and their loved ones are served promptly and understand fully the implications of each service.

The major complaints brought up by families who have experienced disappointments fall into nine categories. Most of them are easily corrected.

1. Visitors are made to feel that they are intruding when in the room with their loved one. Nurses and doctors treat them like impediments in the treatment of their loved one.

   This feeling of intrusion can be easily corrected if you can remember that you are in fact the *employer* of care-givers and have the right and duty to be present on the premises. Simply offer to leave the room during necessary treatment and say that you wish to be called when the treatment is finished. You will find that

77

if you *expect* your desires to be respected, they
will be. And if you enunciate your expectations
firmly and pleasantly, nurses, doctors, and aides
will cooperate with grace.

2. Since private rooms are at a premium and not
    covered by most insurance policies, privacy to
    discuss personal and legal matters is often a
    problem. Privacy can be arranged by asking the
    doctor in charge to arrange for it. Usually he will
    request either a conference room where the
    patient can be taken or a "Do Not Disturb" sign
    that will be honored except for dire emergency
    treatment. Keep your request and the time you
    demand to a minimum.

    Legal papers should be prepared in advance
    and the notary, attorney or witness persuaded
    that a special time slot is available for
    consultation at a specific time and that in the
    interest of your patient's well-being, promptness
    and brevity will be required. (Expect your patient
    to be fatigued and depressed after legal or
    financial discussions and keep these kinds of
    meetings to a minimum.)

3. It is your *right* to be notified promptly if there are
    changes in the patient's condition or if he or she
    has been moved from the assigned room before
    your arrival at the hospital. Unless you have
    experienced the shock of finding an empty bed or
    a stranger where you last saw your loved one,
    you cannot appreciate the importance of
    *immediate notification of change in condition or
    location.* Have your desires here noted on your
    loved one's record and your doctor will
    cooperate.

4. If it has been decided that no extreme measures
    are to be taken to prolong the life of your loved
    one, it is up to you to see that it is prominently
    included in both the doctor's records and the
    hospital records. This is called a "No Code." It is

automatic in hospitals to do everything to maintain life. Their first reaction to a decline in a patient's condition is to put him or her on a life support system. This is as it should be. But when the condition is terminal and you have expressed a desire that nature be allowed to determine the existence of life, foul-ups often occur as doctors try to follow directives in the Living Will. Reaching an understanding with your doctor and other care-givers is the only way to prevent heroic measures from being administered. (See the "Living Will.")

5. If the hospital is unfamiliar to you and/or you are a stranger in the neighborhood, ask for maps and information at the Admittance Desk or go to the Special Services area, the Chaplain's Office, or Hospital Auxiliary for information. Many hospitals provide information on parking, bus routes, and convenient accommodation information along with a brochure which will direct you to eating facilities, the chapel, rest areas, and people who will acquaint you with necessary information for your comfort and convenience. If this information hasn't been provided, *ask* for it.

6. When a patient is admitted to a hospital, it is not unusual for communication with the attending physician to break down. Doctors make their hospital rounds early and late in the day. Your visiting hours and doctor's rounds seldom coincide, which leaves you the alternative of depending on the patient to relay pertinent information on his or her condition or upon the nurses in charge who often (rightly or wrongly) feel it is the doctor's responsibility to give out detailed information to the patient's family. This lack of communication always leads to resentment. If from the outset of hospitalization, you request your doctor to *personally* inform you

79

on the patient's condition and to set up
conferences or telephone calls on a regular basis
at his or her convenience, much unhappiness and
discontent can be eliminated.

7. Misunderstandings of diagnosis and treatment
   also cause apprehension and concern among
   those whose loved one is hospitalized. It comes, I
   think, from the natural assumption on the part of
   the care-givers that we neophytes understand the
   medical terms they use with such facility. We, on
   the other hand, are reluctant to appear ignorant
   or we are in such a state of confusion we can't
   assimilate what we have been told. The result is
   that we either blame the doctor for not telling us
   what we should know, or the doctor is amazed at
   our lack of comprehension. This is when the
   Patient Representative should be contacted.

8. The care of children in the hospital during
   visiting hours can be a problem, especially if you
   live out of town and commute to the hospital. If
   there are no child care facilities in the hospital
   (many have playrooms with attendants), ask the
   social service, special services department, or
   chaplain to find you approved child care service.
   It will eliminate a great deal of stress. The
   welfare of the patient should be paramount in
   considering whether or not a child is allowed
   visiting privileges, and consideration of other
   patients must be emphasized. Rowdy, excited or
   fearful children do not belong in hospital rooms.
   It is unreasonable to expect a small child to
   observe the quiet that should be maintained in a
   hospital. If a child is going to visit a patient, it
   should be understood that the visit will last no
   more than four or five minutes. The best way to
   handle child care is to ask a friend to supervise
   children either at home or in a safe place when
   you go to the hospital.

9. Last but not least are the difficulties one can run

80

into with the hospital's accounting department. If
you have questions concerning your bill or
hospitalization, it is best to speak to the *head* of
the department. Clerks in the accounting division
of the hospital are generally equipped to handle
everyday finances that take place, but a clerk can
seldom handle complicated forms, make
decisions, or understand exceptional problems.
You will save yourself time and frustration if you
go to the top when there are questions or
difficulties.

To sum up the problems and their solutions
regarding hospitals, remember *you are employing
and paying for the services rendered*. It is up to *you*
to let your wishes and needs be known through
the proper channels. If you are not happy with
the service, speak to the doctor. If you are not
satisfied with his response, go up the chain of
command until you are satisfied. Hospitals want
to be of service and to please their clientele.

CHAPTER · 8

Convalescent/ Nursing Homes

One of the most difficult decisions made during a terminal illness involves finding a competent, compassionate and affordable care facility. Most of us depend on recommendations from doctors, friends and clergy, but that is not enough. Before entrusting the care of your loved one to a strange place where he or she will end his/her days, you should become personally acquainted with all aspects of the place, especially with the kind of care that will be given.

With convalescent and nursing homes increasingly under fire for physical, mental, sexual, drug and financial abuses, it is extremely important that any institution your loved one enters should be screened with extreme care.

There are guidelines in almost every state regarding physical layout (fire protection, cleanliness in the kitchen, etc.), but with budget cutbacks, facility administrators are badly overstrained, and in some states, counties, or cities are all but nonexistent. It falls on you to be *the guardian of your patient.*

Because many care facilities pay their staff only minimum wages, patients may receive only minimum care. Attrition is high among the help and often aides are indifferent or indignant.

While this information is grim and not very reassuring, it must be faced and dealt with *before* traumatic problems arise. Carefully researching the place and personnel, and clearly asserting your expectations as to the care and services you require are only the beginning. After checking the certification and credentials of a care facility with the doctor who is caring for your patient, go to the facility and consider the following guidelines before you permit your loved one to enter.

1. Your nose can tell you a great deal about the place. Nursing facilities have to contend with incontinence. The smell of urine or feces, a pile of dirty laundry in the halls, or an overwhelming odor of disinfectant is an indication of problems. Stale cooking odors, dirty dishes on trays or scattered about also tell you something about the housekeeping.
2. Look at the patients who are in bed or in the corridors and recreational rooms. Are they well groomed, dressed cleanly and appropriately, do they seem alert and reasonably happy? Talk to them and *ask questions of them.* If they are evasive, vague, or intimidated or seem overly resentful and aggressive, there may be a reason. Check the place carefully before you admit a patient to its care.
3. Find out how the place controls unruly patients. Drugs? Restraints?
4. What is the ratio of aides and nurses to patients? Are the nurses licensed and registered? Are the aides trained and certified?
5. How often does the doctor *personally* visit the facility? (Frequently, the physician depends on the telephone to check on nursing-home patients.)
6. Are visiting hours strictly enforced or are you allowed to come to the facility when *you* choose? (An open-door policy indicates that the staff is constant in their care of patients.)
7. If possible, get a schedule of routines. How often are patients bathed and groomed? How are they prepared for the night? Who attends to manicures, pedicures, backrubs, etc. Who

dispenses medication? What therapies are available? Are these services a part of the routine or are they extra-charge services?

8. Visit the kitchen. Is there a trained dietician? A good cook? Are the meals balanced and well prepared? Are meals served *hot*, quickly, and pleasing to the eye? Is there enough staff to assist a patient incapable of feeding himself or herself? Try to be at the facility during mealtimes. Know whether the kitchen accommodates those who need special diets. Will they honor a patient's dietary philosophy (vegetarian, religious) and preferences?

9. Are the rooms pleasant, light, airy? Are they clean? Look at baseboards and in corners. Check the toilets and bathrooms for cleanliness and safety bars. Can the patient have a radio, television or tape recorder? Will personal possessions be allowed and will they be secure? (One of the big problems I found in my research was theft.)

10. Interview the director. Research has shown me that there are two categories of nursing-home directors. One is the administrative type who is more involved with the skills of running a smooth operation, keeping expenses in line, dealing with the overwhelming paperwork and personnel problems. The other, for want of a better description, is the hands-on type of administrator who is more patient-involved. This kind of person knows patient needs and names, and works closely with both the family and the care-givers to see that all aspects of care are considered and carried out.

11. What are the costs? There will be additional costs over and above the daily care. Know what they are and who will be responsible for them. Balance the cost against your insurance coverage. Since skilled nursing care is usually covered by

insurance but intermediary care generally is not, it is important that you discuss both, first with your doctor and then with the administrator of the nursing facility. Generally speaking, skilled nursing involves the care of a patient who can be rehabilitated and returned home. Intermediary care is for the chronic or terminally ill, whose chances of being dismissed from the facility in good health are not very good. Insurance coverage, including Medicare, Medicaide, and all the other social insurance, differs widely according to the state in which you live, according to the diagnosis, and according to the terms of care to which you agree. Social workers and administrators of good nursing facilities are aware and helpful in finding a path through "the system" which will benefit the family of the terminally ill and the patient. But remember, it is up to you to examine carefully and fully understand the choices and the services you are buying.

12. Ask about the entertainment, therapy, and recreational programs available. Just knowing they are available to the more ambulatory and less ill will tell you that the nursing home is concerned with the mental and emotional needs of patients.

Next, check references with the following people and places to find out the reputation of the facility.

1. Your doctor. Is he conveniently located to make calls? Has he had other patients in the facility? Does he feel confident that it meets your standards as well as the standards of the county, city and state?

2. Ex-patients and their families. Were they satisfied with the care and treatment?

3. Clergy. What does your priest, rabbi or minister

think about the place? Does he/she call frequently
after visiting hours to know what is happening?

4. The Health and Welfare Departments. Have they
had any complaints? What is the facility's status
in any association it may belong to? How is it
rated by investigation agencies?

5. Medicare, Medicaide, and participating medical
and care-giving coverages. How do the people at
Medicare and/or SSI feel about the place? Any
complaints? DRG (diagnosis-related grouping), for
example, allows only one diagnosis.

6. Better Business Bureau. Any complaints? What is
the credit rating of the facility?

All this takes time and effort but if you are entrusting a
loved one's last days to strangers, you can alleviate much of
the pain of parting by being absolutely certain that you have
given the best by way of care and love in vigilance during
these remaining days.

When you have chosen the care facility and are certain
you have chosen wisely, there are acts of love that will comfort
you and your loved one. First, of course, is a regular schedule
of visits. They need not be prolonged vigils but if you are there
regularly, there will be a sense of security that cannot be
underestimated. If you can, make the patient's space as
personal as possible—with pictures, plants, a favorite blanket
or pillow, his or her favorite scent or cosmetics, a box of mints
or goodies. *Anything* that spells love and caring will add to
the final comfort you can give.

If there seems to be a lack of awareness in the patient,
holding a hand, smoothing a pillow, or speaking of the familiar
somehow makes the patient more comfortable. To make the
final gift, a gift of love is best of all. It will help you meet the
future with the knowledge that you did all you could for the
one you love.

You can receive information and guidelines by writing:

Your state services and facilities
(*See* Yellow Pages)

American Healthcare Association
1200 15th Street
Washington, DC 20005

American College of Nursing Home Administrators
211 E. Chicago Avenue
Chicago, IL 60611

CHAPTER · 9

Home Care

There is no doubt that home is the place one longs for most when one is ill. This is certainly true of the dying. Now, with support systems available to many of us, the wish to be at home among one's loved ones can be a reality. Making the decision to bring the patient home is, of course, very personal and must be measured in terms of capabilities, personalities, and needs. It's a family decision because it is going to be a family project.

At first, the thought of being the primary care-giver when one has no nursing experience is scary, but with information and guidance from trained nurses and doctors, with good home-nursing courses given by community colleges, the Visiting Nurses Association (VNS) and hospice training programs, or in manuals that are clearly written and simple to follow, it can be done.

Home care needs careful preparation. However, with all the health-need equipment available free from agency pools, through rental from surgical supply stores, and with determination, caring for the terminally ill at home is possible.

If the doctor feels it is feasible; if you can get reliable backup help and/or a support group from VNA, hospice, state health system, or a competent health care facility; and if other family members agree that this is what should be, I believe the advantages and pleasures of home care far outweigh any of the difficulties.

One can best base one's judgment on personal experience and the experience of others in the matter of home care. Those with whom I talked found a satisfaction that lasts long, long after death, by caring for their loved one at home in the heart of the family. Each person felt it helped the grieving process after death and healed an accumulation of hurts and guilts that are inevitable in all close relationships. Most felt that the sharing of care and concerns brought family and close friends closer than ever. And although there was admitted fatigue and sorrow, each person who had taken part in home care felt he/she would do it again without hesitation.

Almost everyone mentioned that having the patient at home opened up avenues of communication that were constrained in the hospital, and allowed an intimacy each had longed for. All admitted a certain amount of fear and uncertainty in the undertaking, but said that fear disappeared once they became accustomed to the routine involved in caring for the physical and emotional needs of the patient.

When home care was under the guidance of the Visiting Nurses Association or other home health care organizations that provide round-the-clock consultations and quick response to every emergency, the stress level of family members diminished.

To know that at 2:00 o'clock in the morning or afternoon—whenever help was needed, physical or emotional—one can get a positive and personal response from a caring person familiar with all the ramifications of the illness as well as the emotional and psychological needs of the person taking care of a loved one, and to be sure of positive advice and a willingness to come immediately and evaluate the problem is blessing beyond description. These services are available in every major city and in many communities throughout the country.

Unfortunately, many private home-care services are expensive and not covered by medical insurance policies. However, the place to start, when one has made the decision that home is where the terminally ill will be cared for, is the Visiting Nurses Association or the County Health Services. They know what is available in the community and can explain in detail what you can expect by way of service and cost.

The next step is to investigate the costs involved in home care through your insurance agent. And then balance the cost in money, peace of mind, and your capabilities of home care against the institutional care available to you.

Perhaps a brief personal story will illustrate the ups and downs of home care for the terminally ill. My story began after Bob had been in and out of the hospital for years. He had been in and out of ICU (Intensive Care Unit) many times and it was on a Sunday after one such trip to the hospital that I was with him.

He seemed strangely thoughtful and quiet, and I waited for him to tell me what was troubling him. Finally he said, "Norm, I've got to tell you that I've come to a couple of conclusions." I waited. He went on, "You know, hospitals are great. They are geared to make people well. They just *won't* let you die. I'm so *damned* tired of being poked and prodded and piped! Please, can I come home and rest? I know it's not going to be easy, but I'll do my damndest not to be a problem. I want to see the river and be with our things and see the kids and you in our own home."

I fought to keep tears from falling. "But what will Dr. H——— say? Will they let you out? Do you *really* think we can do it?"

He pushed himself up in bed a little and said, "Look, this isn't a prison! I signed myself in, I can sign myself out! If Dr. H——— doesn't like it, to hell with him! I *really* want to get the show on the road."

We made plans and I left the hospital scared out of my wits. I had no nursing experience other than the normal child-caring jobs that come with motherhood. On the way home I counted my assets in nursing and found that they numbered three. I could take temperatures, I could make beds, and *probably* bathe Bob—sort of.

I decided that if Bob was going to be at home, the logical place for him would be in the living room. If he was there, he could see the river (we lived in a houseboat on the Columbia River), watch television, hear his music, and watch the fireplace. It would be more pleasant for him to be in the heart of things, near the kitchen and dining room. He could visit with friends more comfortably than if he was isolated in the bedroom, and it would be convenient for me to be close to him. That night I rearranged the living room with the help of one of my sons.

Next morning I called an oxygen rental place which had furnished us with a portable oxygen machine, and they promptly delivered a big blue tank with instructions on its use. I borrowed a wheelchair from a neighbor to bring Bob from the car down the ramp to our houseboat; another friend had a rubberized draw sheet and a foam mattress designed to keep patients from getting bedsores, which hospital beds had given Bob, and a sheepskin mat that would also help in that area. There was an abundance of those plastic basins, cups, and stuff that come in plastic bags given to us whenever Bob had gone into the hospital before, along with the bottles of lotion and mouthwash. I would have access to a portable toilet and bedpan when we needed them. I made up his bed and went to the supermarket to shop for his favorite foods and a little before noon, I went to the hospital.

Bob was waiting to start for home. He said he had told the doctors how he felt and that they had said they "hoped" we knew what we were doing! We bade farewell to his roommate and the nurses and thanked everyone for their kindness, and with my heart in my mouth we left. Bob sensed my trepidation and when we got to a stop light, he reached over and patted my hand. "You'll do just fine, darling! Ain't nobody can take better care of me in the whole world!" He sighed. "God, it's good to be *out!*"

I began to feel more optimistic. If he was going to die, and reality told me he was, the least I could do was to care for him and fulfill his wishes. "Please, God, help us."

I managed the wheelchair down the ramp and even navigated through the doorway and hall to the living room. We worked together to get him into bed and he lay back, closed his eyes and said, "This is it! This is *perfect!* Thank you," and fell asleep. That was how it began and that was how it ended, with Bob sleeping quietly in the place he loved best.

My employers were most kind in allowing me to take a leave of absence. Our family and friends rallied round and gave of themselves in making those last four months more comfortable, natural and happy. Bob helped me with the intricacies of his support machines and told me that bathing him would be no different than washing the car. "You do one fender at a time!" He cheered me on when I tried and valiantly put up with me when I bungled.

Caring for him became easier than I thought it would be because of his never-failing humor. He directed and I performed. As he became weaker and I became more tired and sorrowful, others came to help. If I were to list the people and kindnesses, they would fill a book. If I could explain the advantages and relief of joining him in his care during this last period of his life, I would be a master writer.

At the time he came home, there was no hospice program, no support groups here, and we were out of the area served by the Visiting Nurses Association, so we had to wing it. Now things have changed and both the hospice program and VNA are available to my neighbors. I know that if I had been able to call on them, life would have been still easier. The point is we made it. It isn't impossible for anyone who really wants to have home care to carry it out. I know I would do it again without hesitation. You don't have to be brave, only determined.

When one has decided on home care for the terminally ill, it is vital to begin with a *plan*. Home care means 24-hour-a-day concern. The needs of the patient are of prime consideration, but the needs of the care-giver, the family and all those who will be impacted or involved should be carefully thought out before one brings a patient home.

A flexible but daily routine should be considered. This plan needs to start with basic patient care. Medication at set times. Baths and grooming within, say, a 2-hour span. Meals planned and served at regular hours. A specific day for haircuts, shampoos, pedicures, manicures and massages. Periods of rest for both the patient and the care-giver. There must be days when a care-giver can get away from the house and do something pleasant and unrestricted.

Visiting hours when a patient is at home can become a problem unless consideration and assertion are combined to protect the strength of the patient and the sanity of the caregiver. If, from the time you are contemplating home care, you do not make it abundantly clear in a firm but pleasant way that the only way you will be able to cope with the responsibilities is by maintaining a routine, *and ask for assistance and cooperation* from family and friends, you will find yourself being nurse, hostess, telephone answering service and chief cook and bottle washer.

I handled it well for us, I think, by pulling out the plug on the telephone from 9 to 11 A.M., which was bathing, laundry, special medication, bed changing and cleaning up time. From 11 till 12 was lunch (actually the heaviest meal of the day) and the afternoon was then free from 1 to 4:30 or 5 when Bob was delighted to have visitors. This was when I put on a pot of coffee, put cups on the counter and wine in the cooler, and left him and his family, friends and neighbors to their own devices while I ran errands, made phone calls upstairs, or got away from it all with a book, a rest period or a bubble bath. No one seemed to object to my absence from the sick room, and it did wonders for my perspective. After all, Bob was the focal point of the visits, not me. People who knew us realized that they were giving both of us a loving gift by accepting our routine as a natural course of events. Being *maitre d'* of the sick room is not part of the bargain in home care.

With a *stated* routine and a flexible approach to everything other than medication, patient care and voicing your needs, you can achieve happier and more relaxed days for everyone in the family and help maintain equilibrium.

Home care, Visiting Nurses, County Health Services, and Out-Patient Social Workers will generally tell you what you will need by way of equipment to make a patient comfortable and make your work easier.

It's the better part of wisdom to ask for help and advice until you have learned how to care for someone confined to bed. The techniques are really quite simple, and once you learn how, for instance, to lift a patient, change a bed with someone in it, and give a bath the proper way, your confidence will soar and the satisfaction of knowing you have the skills to help someone you love will bring you a sense of security and satisfaction you'll never forget.

The people who rent or lend equipment give explicit directions on usage. The home-care personnel will tell you what you need and they, too, will show you how to use any necessary equipment, what to do under various circumstances, and whom to call if there are problems.

When a patient must be monitored 24 hours a day and the amount of time for home-care assistance must be limited, choose the period for outside help when you need a rest.

My choice would have been from midnight so that I might have had uninterrupted nights' sleep. As it was, my sleep pattern was disturbed to the extent that it took almost a year to reestablish a 6- to 8-hour span of uninterrupted rest, and that rest was sorely needed when I was trying to reestablish my life after Bob died.

Equipment Helpful in Caring for a Person Who Is Ill

Hospital bed (can be rented)
Foam mattress (surgical or hospital supply store)
Wheelchair (can be rented or borrowed)
Raised toilet seat fixture, if ambulatory (surgical or hospital supply store)
Portable toilet (can be rented)
Bedpan or urinal (drugstore or hospital supply store)
Rubber sheets (hospital supply store)
Flannel draw sheets (hospital supply store)
Thermometer
Bed tray (can be rented)
Terrycloth or flannel bath sheets (easy to make, or use large beach towel)
Bathtub stool (surgical supply store)
Shower extension (hardware or drugstore)
Bath rail (drugstore)
Hoyer lifts (can be rented)
Fleece pad (hospital or surgical supply store)
Oxygen (can be rented)
Commercial-strength spray deodorizer
Special medicated toilet tissue
Massage lotion (backrubs and massages soothe muscular cramps and are relaxing)
Talc, creams, body lotions
Mouthwash and swabs
Bell or intercom system

Most of these things can be purchased from any major catalog store, such as Sears or Montgomery Ward.

Questions to Consider in Hiring Home-Care Givers

1. What is the care-givers' training in patient care?
2. Are they licensed and bonded?
3. Are they legally able to give shots and drugs?
4. Are they familiar with the use of necessary equipment?
5. Are they and their care covered by insurance?
6. What is the cost per hour?
7. What is the extent of the care to be given? Bathing? Grooming? Included or extra cost?
8. Is transportation an additional cost?
9. Is simple meal preparation included?
10. Do they have references? (Check them.)

In a pre-care interview with care-givers, one should focus on the concerns and the expectations of both the care-givers and family—the patient should be included in deciding whom to hire. This relationship between care-giver, patient, and family is going to be sensitive and intimate. Careful choices should be paramount and these are some of the subjects that should be clearly discussed and decided upon in addition to the previous ten points.

1. What to expect regarding meals and snacks for the care-giver.
2. Social telephone calls of the care-giver.
3. Sleep and rest periods of the care-giver.
4. Days off.
5. Room care for the patient—dusting, vacuuming, neatness, etc.
6. Patient's laundry needs.
7. Breaks or periods of relief for the care-giver during intensive care.
8. Idiosyncrasies or eccentricities of the patient and any other different or difficult situations to be met.

CHAPTER · *10*

Hospices

The hospice concept of care for the terminally ill has long been practiced in Europe and has been gaining enthusiastic acceptance in the United States during the past decade. With life-prolonging medicine and procedures there came an awareness that the special needs of the dying could best be met under special conditions and outside the parameters of ordinary hospital or nursing home care.

Facilities which would support the comfort of patient and family in both physical and intangible ways during the last months of life are promoted in an environment geared toward making this final illness a cooperative effort between care-givers, family and patient. The basic characteristics of a hospice program as defined by the American Cancer Society is a "program of coordinated out- and in-patient services primarily concerned with home care, with back-up in-patient services when home care is not feasible."

There are five kinds of hospice care available in many areas of the country:

1. The free-standing hospice. This is an entity of its own rather like a nursing or convalescent facility, but it operates solely for the care of the terminally ill.
2. The hospital-affiliated, free-standing hospice. This is connected with a hospital but has a separate building or wing in which it cares for patients with an independent staff.
3. The hospital-based hospice. This type would have

a centralized palliative care or hospice unit or a hospice team which visits patients. It might also have units which are operated as a part of the Health Maintenance Organization within the hospital.

4. The hospice within an extended care facility (convalescent) or nursing home.

5. The Home-Care Hospice Program. This may be hospital-based, nursing home-based, or community-based and visits the home of the terminally ill for as long as it is feasible.

These are but five of many variations found in hospice care throughout the country. What all hospice treatment facilities have in common is the goal not to save or prolong a patient's life but to help patients live out their time with dignity and to make them as comfortable as possible within the limits of the illness.

In some places the visiting Nurses Association works closely with the hospice in evaluating the patient's and family's needs and in administering such drugs and treatments that by law only an RN or MD are allowed to give. The hospice nurse is always in contact with your doctor.

Members of the hospice team may include home health aides, social workers, physical therapists, speech therapists, occupational therapists, and hospital assistants depending on the patient's needs and the doctor's orders. There may also be a respite team to relieve the prime care-giver for a few hours or days so that he/she can get rest and regain perspective.

The home health aide may give baths, shampoos, and general grooming assistance, prepare meals, help with errands or carry out simple nursing procedures by instructions of the nurse. Some will help with light housekeeping and cooking.

Social workers are available to discuss your present and future concerns. He or she will help you with decisions regarding treatment and will help you find available community resources and can discuss any problems concerning medical bills, insurance problems, and the like. They specialize in lightening the burden of terminal illness in today's society.

Total patient care includes dealing with family and other important relationships. Emotional assistance is given to both the patient and those closest to him or her, and spiritual concerns are appropriately met. Pain, nausea and vomiting are as effectively controlled as much as possible. Health care is under the direction of qualified physicians; interdisciplinary needs such as social services, therapies, consultations and pastoral care are available.

Professional care is augmented by carefully selected, fully trained volunteers. The services of a hospice are available 'round the clock and are dedicated to the well-being of the patient and his loved ones. These services extend beyond the death of the patient to help families through bereavement and rehabilitation of the family unit. Hospice services are based on need rather than on ability to pay.

Hospice Criteria and Standards

The National Hospice Organization has developed twenty-two standards and criteria to describe hospice care and programs. Those standards are detailed in "The Standards of a Hospice Program of Care," a NHO document that serves as the basis for accrediting hospice programs. The most important criteria are listed below:

- Palliative care is the most important form of care when cure is no longer possible.
- The goal of palliative care is the prevention of distress from chronic signs and symptoms.
- Admission to a hospice program of care is dependent on patient and family needs and their expressed request for care.
- Hospice care consists of a blending of professional and nonprofessional services.
- Hospice care considers all aspects of the lives of patients and their families as valid areas of therapeutic concern.
- Hospice care is respectful of all patient and family belief systems, and will employ resources to meet the

98

personal, philosophical, moral, and religious needs of patients and their families.

- A hospice care program considers the patient and the family together as the unit of care. (Hospice personnel realize everyone closely related to the patient is suffering and may require assistance of one kind or another.)
- Hospice care programs seek to identify, coordinate, and supervise persons who can give care to patients who do not have a family member available to take on the responsibility of giving care.
- Hospice care for the family continues into the bereavement period.
- Hospice care is available twenty-four hours a day, seven days a week.
- Hospice care is provided by an interdisciplinary team.
- The optional control of distressful symptoms is an essential part of a hospice care program requiring medical, nursing, and other services of the interdisciplinary team.
- The hospice care team will have a medical director on staff and a working relationship with the patient's physician.
- Based on the patient's needs and preferences as determining factors on the setting and location for care, a hospice program provides in-patient care and care in the home setting.

* * *

At present there are over 1,300 hospice programs in operation throughout the country and more are being formed to meet the needs of patients and families who feel that quality time for the incurably ill is a noble and compassionate way to end life. Thus far the emphasis seems to be on cancer victims with a prognosis of six months of life, but it is the hope of hospice supporters that other kinds of terminal patients will soon be able to take advantage of the services they offer. There are now hospice programs for victims of AIDS.

While doing research for this book I couldn't help but be

a bit envious of those who are using the hospice program. So many times during my husband's final illness the services they offer during the last months of life would have been such a help to both of us. If you and your loved one have decided that home is where he or she wishes to spend these last days, I strongly urge you to seek out and support the hospice programs in your community.

For further information regarding hospice and the address of hospice programs near you, write to:

National Hospice Organization
1311-A Dolly Madison Blvd.
McLean, VA 22101
(703) 356-6770

CHAPTER · **11**

Help for the Bills

One of the least known and understood laws passed by the federal government is the Hill-Burton Act (1946), which provides aid for hospital construction and modernization. This act and subsequent regulations require hospitals receiving federal aid to provide services to everyone regardless of race, creed or color, and to provide a reasonable amount of free or low-cost care to patients unable to pay.

Under further regulations issued by the U.S. Department of Health and Human Services, hospitals must (1) provide free care equal to ten percent of their grant or three percent of their operating costs; (2) use uniform eligibility standards for free or low-cost services; (3) give patients individual written notice of this; and (4) keep separate financial records on Hill-Burton cases for public inspection.

Hospitals must, under the Hill-Burton act, provide emergency services (not necessarily free services) to anyone living or working in their service area and must not use exclusionary admission policies such as requiring a deposit or accepting only patients referred by doctors with hospital privileges.

For further information:
  U.S. Public Health and Human Services
  Washington, D.C. 20201
Or read this book:
  Advocate's Guide to Hill-Burton Uncompensated and Community Clearinghouse
  Clearinghouse Review

500 N. Michigan Avenue, Suite 940
Chicago, Illinois 60611

Laws and rules change rapidly and vary from state to state. Federal rulings, especially in social issues, are not only changing but being reinterpreted on all levels. What may have been true for a friend or neighbor last year will not necessarily hold true for you.

Consulting with a lawyer, certified tax consultant, Social Services administrator and others who deal on a daily basis with current rulings and laws will save you time, energy and money. Every city, county and state has agencies geared to help you. They can be located by contacting:

Dept. of Health, Education and Welfare
Washington, D.C. 20208

Ask them for assistance in finding competent, affordable assistance in your area of concern (legal, medical, tax information, Social Security benefits, etc.).

Your state's Attorney General is also able and willing to direct you to helpful agencies. If you are having difficulties with a particular agency, do not hesitate to inform your political representatives of your needs—they understand the formula for getting through the complexities of government systems and bureaucracies.

PART·THREE

Legalities and Decisions

CHAPTER · 12

Very Important Papers

When I realized that Bob's illness was not a passing thing and that life was going to radically change, I was face to face with the truth that we had lived without giving a great deal of thought to death or providing for each other after death. Oh yes, we had insurance—the kind that would take care of the children and me if Bob died while they were young. We had invested in the future we both assumed we would share and had not given much thought to either of us being left alone. It was a foolish assumption, but in our case I had never known life without Bob and he had never been without me somewhere in his life. The idea of life without him was as unthinkable as living without hands, feet or heart. We had made our wills with the children in mind and that was that.

Common sense should have told me that if Bob died, I would not follow suit or cease to exist. It was not until I took a part-time job in a legal firm that I realized the value of an up-to-date will and the complications that not having one brings to survivors. I was reluctant and embarrassed to bring up the subject of our unrealistic approach in ways I never would have been had Bob been healthy. Somehow it felt terribly inappropriate to say to someone you loved so much, "Hey, fellow, you and I have goofed on the subject of—what? Dying and surviving? Providing for each other? Facing the facts of life and death? There seemed to be no way I could talk about the subject of wills and powers of attorney without

feeling that I had given up hope of his recovery and admit defeat.

I thought about asking the boys to approach the subject to their Dad, but that was a cop-out. I thought about having Bob read some sort of article about the need for having one's estate in order, but I knew he wouldn't, because by this time he was reading only escape books and occasionally the newspaper. And so I batted ploys and plans around ad nauseum until it occurred to me that Bob was as guilty as I in not having prepared for the future. Simple as that! I would admit my own failure and assume he would agree we both had been remiss.

It was amazing how casual the conversation was. I said something like, "You know, it occurred to me that if I got knocked off traveling to work, you'd be up the creek as far as property and stuff is concerned. I'm going to make an appointment to have a current will drawn up for us and we'll get a couple of neighbors to witness it and that at least will be settled." All he said was, "OK, it sounds like a good idea, but for Pete's sake drive carefully—I don't want you 'knocked off.' "

I had two simple wills drawn up with room for an addendum in case either of us wanted to add anything, and two Power of Attorney forms (one for each of us). We invited two friends to witness (one of whom was a Notary Public). After we signed we celebrated with a glass of wine.

Doing all you can do for someone you love brings peace. We never discussed either of those documents again. They were kept in our lawyer's office with copies in our safety deposit box. The lesson I learned was that if I was casual, honest and sharing, we could handle sensitive areas that should be covered sooner rather than later. From then on it was easier to say, "Don't you think it would be a good idea to have this or that item of property put into survivorship?" The answer is always "Yes."

Chances are you will need the advice and/or guidance of an attorney now or in the near future. Most people chose an attorney on the recommendation of a friend or their banker. *Always ask for an estimate of costs* for an attorney's work. If

he/she states the charge is hourly, ask how many hours the job will take. If the charges are too high, call Legal Aid, your local Human Resources Department, or ask your clergy to help you find competent legal help within your ability to pay.

By the end of this year or this illness, you will need an accountant, tax consultant or good bookkeeper. No matter how you may pride yourself in your ability to balance a budget, keep the accounts, or fill out tax forms, when you are under stress, terribly busy, extremely tired and experiencing an entirely new way of life, you will need back-up help in accounting. Often there is one member of the family or close friend who will be willing to take care of accounting—at least to the extent of balancing the checkbook, writing checks for you to sign, filing the bills, filling out insurance claims and stashing away the piles of receipts for parking, gas, prescriptions, photocopying, and similar items that you will learn are important for tax purposes. (During the last year of Bob's illness, I collected two shopping bags full of that sort of stuff, all very important at tax time.)

A tax accountant and an attorney are tax deductible expenses. While they may seem expensive at the time (remember, you should find out before hiring them how expensive they will be), they have the know-how and perspective to handle with ease the sort of thing you will find unbearably confusing during this time. Also, having these things handled by a professional gives credibility to your tax returns.

Your attorney will tell you which important forms should be filled out to help in the orderly transfer of property should the need arise. Although you may feel least able to cope, it is most important for you to know and understand your financial and legal position. It is when you are feeling most scatterbrained with stress that you will be asked to produce certificates, documents and records you delegated to the bottom drawer of your desk or tossed in a safety deposit box long ago.

The strongest argument for putting your paper world in order as soon as possible is that you will probably need the help of the ill person to locate and explain certain important records, directions, names, papers or items that only he or she can help you with. Taking care of these matters *now*, while

your loved one is coherent and capable of making rational decisions, will give you the time you need to deal with more abstract, important personal issues that will arise. Dealing *now* with legal proofs of birth, academia, military service, marriage, divorce, finances and properties can make the difference between handling present and future affairs smoothly or going through the hellish nightmare "the system" can inflict on survivors because they didn't know, didn't care, or didn't understand. Some of these legal proofs and information will be needed early on in an illness, some will be important during the more critical times and many will be vital after the illness has been resolved. In any event, each of us owes it to our loved ones to leave important records in good order.

Because there are no national standards for handling transfers of properties, Wills, Living Wills, Trusts, Power of Attorney, etc., we felt it important to include all the possible records you might need for your files. A clear photocopy is generally adequate as legal proof, allowing the original to remain secure in a safety deposit box. Sample copies of Power of Attorney, Will, Donor Form, Living Will, etc. are shown here merely as *examples* of the type of legal documents you may need to produce in order to avoid controversy and stalemates in the legal process. *Since each state has its own requirements, it is important that you know and abide by the legal requirements of the state in which you reside.* An attorney, paralegal, library or legal-business stationery outlet are good sources for the forms and information required in your location.

If you do not have any of the informational records which follow, a simple letter requesting that it be sent to you and a self-addressed stamped envelope is usually all that is necessary.

Sample
Your Address

To Whom It May Concern:

Please send me a photocopy of (*document and name*) which should be in your records dated _____.

108

Enclosed you will find a self-addressed stamped envelope. If there is a charge for this service, please submit a bill with this photocopy and I will send you a check by return mail.

Thank you sincerely,

Your Name

The following list of VIPs (Very Important Papers) should see you through any eventuality in which legal proof is required. Wherever possible, directions or addresses have been included. Don't bother organizing them now, just put them in an envelope or box and index them later. The important thing for now is to have all of these papers in one place.

(VIPs) Very Important Papers

See Appendix I for Sample Forms (page 169).

1. *Record of birth. Birth certificate* or baptismal certificate or, if you have neither, write to U.S. Commerce Department, Bureau of Census requesting an *Application for Search of Census Records* (cost $4.00) or write to the Records Department of city, county or state, giving full name (maiden name in case of a married woman), place and date of birth.
If none of the above verifications are available, these records are usually acceptable. You will need at least *three* of these:
School records
Marriage certificate
Citizenship papers
Military records
Life insurance policy
Family Bible
2. *Marriage certificate.* May be obtained by writing city, county or state for photocopy or ask for church photocopy (diocesan records are also available in Catholic or Episcopalian churches).

109

3. *Social Security number.* If the Social Security card is not available, look at the W-2 IRS form and verify the number on it by calling your nearest Social Security Office.
4. *Divorce papers.* Verify with photocopies from Department of Records (Vital Statistics) of the city, county and/or state in which it took place.
5. Names of *children* (and grandchildren), along with addresses. If you will be applying for aid to dependent children, you will also need their birth certificates.
6. Names of *brothers and sisters* of patient, with addresses.
7. Names of *parents* (including mother's maiden name) and addresses.
8. *Military discharge papers* and other military records can be found by contacting the Veterans Administration. Note citations, honors and medals for the record.
9. You will need to have *current tax forms* (state and federal) for at least the past three years, along with photocopies of W-2 forms.
10. *Titles of ownership*—house, property, vehicles, etc. (keep originals in safety deposit box and photocopies for records). See attorney if there are any questions as to inheritance.
11. *Current contracts* (mortgage and time purchases). *Check to see if there is a disability or a life insurance policy* attached to these contracts.
12. *Insurance policies*—name of company, type of policy, name and address of agent and number on policy.
13. *Job title*, name and address of employer and name of immediate supervisor and telephone numbers.
14. All *benefits and contracts* (stock options, insurance policies, union benefits, etc.) at place of employment.
15. *Checking and savings accounts*—IRA, Keogh

Mutual funds, special accounts, savings
certificates (photocopy for files).

16. *Brokerage firm*—name, broker account number,
telephone number. Copy of transaction records.
17. *Safety deposit box* number and location of key.
Who has a duplicate key?
18. All *partnership papers*, business contracts, and
agreements (photocopy for files).
19. *Will*—location of original and photocopy. (See
page 173 for sample.)
20. *Executor or trustee*—name, address and
relationship.
21. *Living Will*—photocopies to go to doctor, hospital,
next of kin, executor, attorney and one kept in
record file. (See page 170 for sample.)
22. *Letter of Intent*—original should be readily
available in a safe place and photocopy in file
folder. (See page 171 for sample.)
23. *Power of Attorney*—photocopies for doctor, lawyer,
next of kin, and file folder. (See page 172 for
sample.)
24. *Organ Donor forms*—photocopies to doctor,
attorney, next of kin. Obtained from hospital,
university medical school or specific support
organization (heart, lung, kidney, eye
foundations).
25. Explicit directions as to *disposition of remains*
unless so stated in Letter of Intent. Photocopies to
doctor, attorney, next of kin. Cremation and
burial forms available. (See page 123 for sample.)
Funeral or memorial service desired.
26. *Medicare, Medicaide*—medical numbers if
applicable, photocopies to doctor, hospital,
attorney and next of kin.
27. *Personal reference file* should include:
Church/religious affiliations
Professional affiliations
Social and civic memberships
Offices and honors

      Schools and colleges, dates and degrees
      Names of family members and close friends
      Favorite charities

28. *Credit card names and numbers.* Be sure to have credit cards recorded in both your names if married so that credit is established in case of the death of either spouse.

At this time, it would be a good idea to call your utility company to be certain that your telephone, electric, gas, water, and other utilities are also in *both* names so that there will be no disconnect and reconnect charges in case of the death of one spouse or partner.

This file will be a valuable tool in dealing with attorneys, estate planners, probate, newspapers, media articles or obituaries.

Getting all the vital statistics organized and out of the way when you are under stress is not easy but the rewards in peace of mind are worth every minute. You will have prepared yourself and your family for all known contingencies and will have removed many of the greatest frustrations that haunt the latter stages of a terminal illness and the early phases of grief—times when you are least able to think rationally. Equally important, you will have given your loved one the opportunity to make decisions about the disposition of material property, which are rightfully his or hers to make.

Survivorship and Joint Ownership

Survivorship and joint ownership does not negate the need for a will but it does simplify matters in the handling of finances, taxes and property. By placing all property in survivorship and all utility bills, insurance policies, credit cards, and such in two names, one can usually avoid the expense and confusion often associated with the business aspects of handling a terminal illness and the legal and financial difficulties that come with the death of a spouse or parent.

Homes, cars, boats and other personal properties can be put in joint ownership in most places by simply stating one's wishes to the proper local or state authorities, and adding names to existing titles. Stocks, bonds, annuities and trusts can be changed from one owner to survivor or joint ownership by a simple signature on a proper form. Savings accounts, checking accounts and safety deposit boxes are also handled by proper forms and witnessed signatures.

The important thing to remember is that these things should be done at the earliest possible date. They will help clarify your position now and be of tremendous value in the future. You will save attorney fees by taking care of seemingly insignificant items *now*, for regardless of the outcome of this illness, you will have a clearly defined picture of your assets and liabilities.

An example of what can happen if only one name appears on the household utilities may be appropriate here. Say husband, wife and children live in one household. Husband placed his signature only on the connect orders of telephone, electricity, gas and water. Husband also has the sole valid signature on several credit cards. Husband writes the checks and the savings account is in his name alone. If Husband dies without Wife's name being registered as survivor or joint owner on these various utility and financial documents, she will, in many states, have to pay sizable amounts of money to have the utilities "reconnected" in her name (utility companies say the cost of "reconnect" is to pay for the paperwork involved. The cost can be in the hundreds of dollars). As for family finances, in some states it will take months for the legal system to turn the money in his checking account over to her. The same thing is true of stocks, bonds and certificates. What may have been an acceptable manner of handling family finances while both Husband and Wife were in good health can become a nightmare and a bitter memory during illness or after death. Sharing financial responsibility before a crisis strikes makes it possible to carry on during the crisis without panic.

Transferring Titles

Transferring titles on personal property is one way to eliminate legal hassles in the event of the death of a mate or partner.

Most automobile, boat, and airplane titles have an assignment form on the back. This assignment of title is required for a new title to be issued. The enclosed form Assignment of Title is standard and acceptable in most states. The Motor Vehicle Department, an attorney, or a paralegal can verify its legality wherever you live. (See page 169 for sample Assignment of Title.)

Keeping Records

Tax laws change rapidly and even the rules and regulations which have been standard for many years are often interpreted in different ways by different tax accountants. The only way to receive tax benefits by way of deductions is to keep records and receipts. This does not have to be a precise job, but it does require a certain amount of discipline. Save all receipts! Record all expenses. Date everything. I found a small pocket calendar was an invaluable tool for keeping track of daily expenses. I could jot down those items for which I had no receipt and tuck the receipts I did have in the pages until Monday rolled around (the day I set aside for paperwork) and could file them properly.

When you realize that the following items are only a *few* tax deductible items connected with an illness, you begin to see why a simple method of keeping track of all expenses can be important.

Abdominal supports/back supports, etc. (prescribed)
Acupuncture
Ambulance
Anesthetist
Braces
Cardiographs
Chiropodist
Chiropractor
Christian Science Practitioners (authorized)
Convalescent home (medical treatment only)

Dental services
Dentures
Dermatologist
Equipment for the sick room that is prescribed (rented or purchased)
Eyeglasses
Food or beverages prescribed in addition to regular diet (get statement from doctor)
Gifts of clothing or furniture to charitable

114

non-profit organizations
Gynecologist
Hearing aid and batteries
Home changes or
alterations such as ramps,
hoists, etc. (should be
verified)
Home health services of
many kinds
Insulin treatment
Hospital expenses
Invalid chair
Lab tests
Medications prescribed by
doctor
Nursing services (including
room and board if
provided)
Occupational therapy
Ophthalmologist
Optician
Optometrist
Oral surgery
Osteopath (licensed)
Pacemaker
Physical exams

Physical therapist
Physician
Psychiatrist
Psychologist
Psychotherapy
Radiation therapy as well
as other chemotherapies
Restraining equipment
Speech therapy
Sick room supplies and
equipment
Telephone calls connected
with illness
Telephone equipment for
handicapped
Transportation expenses
for medical purposes
(parking, tolls, taxi and
bus fares)
Vaccines
Vitamins prescribed by
doctor
Wheelchairs
Whirlpool bath equipment
(prescribed)

Some of these expenses will be totally covered, some partially covered and some not covered by insurance. It is important to keep all of the records and total costs so that your tax preparer can figure out and utilize all the tax advantages to which you are entitled.

Our accountant suggested that I divide the expenses connected with Bob's illness into three categories: (1) medical (doctor's bills, prescriptions, equipment, etc.), (2) hospital (itemized bills submitted by the hospital to the insurance company), and (3) miscellaneous (telephone bills, transportation, parking, home aids such as an intercom, and anything having to do with Bob's care and comfort). I put these expenses into a large brown envelope along with a list of expenses I had jotted down on my calendar (pay phone calls, parking meter costs, mileage to and from the doctor's or hospital) and when it was tax time, I turned these bulky envelopes over to the accountant, who had more knowledge, experience and patience than I to figure them out. I was amazed at how seemingly insignificant daily expenses connected with Bob's illness mounted up over the months.

To feel that you must *personally* do the complicated bookwork involved in figuring out income tax is self-defeating. Your job right now is to delegate complicated areas of your life to experts whom you can trust to handle the financial and legal problems with dispatch and expertise. Their work for you is also a tax deduction.

Before you hire a lawyer or tax accountant check his or her credentials if he or she is unknown to you through the professional organizations (American Bar Association and/or Certified Public Accountant Organization or through your bank manager) and be certain to ask him or her to give you a written estimate of the cost you should expect for his services. If you are low on funds, or if there is any doubt that you can pay these people immediately and in full for their services, make financial arrangements *before* you hire them to work for you. As a final bit of advice, ask in advance of your appointment what documentation and records they will need. Remember, time is money. At a time when legal charges can cost between $50 to $200 an hour, you can see why having all the information they will need on hand can work to your advantage.

Wills

Every adult should have a will and it should be written by an attorney.

A will is primarily written for the orderly disposition of the property and possessions of the person for whom it is written. If a person dies without a will, he is determined to be *intestate* and his choice in the matter of disposition is taken away and given to the state in which he resided prior to his death; his estate will be disposed of according to the laws of that state.

To have a will written by an attorney is not usually expensive. The Legal Aid Society, State Bar Association or your banker can give you the name of a competent attorney who will tell you the exact cost for this service. A sample of the general form of a Last Will and Testament is found in Appendix I on page 173. This is only a guide to familiarize you with its coverage.

Each state's laws vary in signing procedures, numbers of witnesses, and the like, but all attorneys will need certain information before writing a will; by having that information readily available you will save both time and money. If you have gathered up all the Very Important Papers, it will simplify the process considerably. Most attorneys want the following information:

1. Real estate
2. Personal effects
3. Savings and checking accounts
4. Stocks, bonds and certificates and any other property owned by the person who will be signing the Will

This list and the names of those to whom these properties will go is usually all that is required. However, if it is desired, an executor or trustee can be named by the writer of the Will and can be directed to sell all properties and dispense the proceeds to specific recipients.

Wills can be simple or complicated depending on the wishes of its signer. The important thing is that everyone should have one which is up-to-date and valid in the state in which he or she resides.

Finances

Unless you're a real feather-head or a happy-go-lucky billionaire you are bound to be worried about finances when someone you love is dying. The cost of medical and hospital care in this country is a perpetual nightmare. However, there are some things you can do to help protect your assets from the hungry maws of the health system—and it is imperative that you begin as soon as possible.

Know Your Assets

Do not delay for one moment finding out exactly what your family owns, how much it is worth, how much money is in your savings and checking accounts, etc. A list of the important information you must have is included (see page 117 of this section).

Know Your Expenses

Know how much you should expect this illness to cost. Good published guidelines exist on the approximate cost of almost every disease known to mankind. Insurance companies, the Health, Education and Welfare Dept., and social service agencies depend on these financial projections in factoring the costs of their services. Hospitals know almost to the penny the cost of each bed, each treatment and therapy; they know to the milligram the cost of medication. The administration (or perhaps the chaplain) of the institution should know or can find out the approximate cost of any illness.

When your doctor talks about medication and/or treatment, *ask how much it will cost*. Do not blindly accept any and all treatments without knowing the cost. Do not allow your physicians to remain aloof to the cost of what he/she is prescribing. If this is in fact a *terminal* illness, the emphasis should be placed on comfort of body and mind. The stress of the high costs of prolongation should not be added to an already overburdened family.

Your medical/hospital insurance will pay a certain percentage of costs. Find out *exactly* how much, the limitations of expense, and how much of the cost you will be expected to pay. Brace yourself! This will be depressing news.

Know What You Can Expect

When you know the average cost of the illness you are facing, it is *imperative* that you learn *immediately* how to protect your assets from depletion or confiscation brought about by catastrophic medical costs. Get the advice of a competent attorney or tax consultant who is conversant with state laws on transferring property and/or placing it beyond the reach of creditors. Almost every state has sheltering or protective laws in force if only you know how to use them. The quicker you act to find out what to expect, the better your protection will be.

Know Where to Go for Help

When bills mount up and you know you will not be able to pay them immediately, go to the manager of your creditor's Accounting Department (don't discuss the problem at the clerk's desk—insist on seeing the manager or head accountant). Explain the situation and assure him you will do whatever you can to pay your bill. *Do not* sign a note or any loan form which requires interest. Give yourself time to think out the ways and means of payment *before* you commit yourself to any financial arrangements. Talk over these arrangements with an expert.

If your creditors are adamant, threatening or uncooperative about payments, take your financial problems to Consumer Credit counselors (non-profit) and let them help you with the problem. If there is a legal problem, Legal Aid or the State Bar Association will be able to help you. If you need a representative to help you with your problem, ask your rabbi, priest, minister or an attorney to speak for you.

Know What You Are Buying

Do not meekly accept any and all patient treatments and therapies your doctors may offer without questioning the cost. Remember that while you may feel the sky should be the limit in the care and treatment of your loved one, reality demands limits to what can be spent. If the disease is terminal, if you will be burdened for decades to come (and many people find themselves in that position), if you will be jeopardizing the stability of your family, think long and hard about unproven, unnecessary, unjustified prolongation and/or uncomfortable extra treatments. Allow the patient to decide on crucial treatments and how much he/she is willing to spend after *all* the facts are clearly defined and the consequences considered.

119

Know the Law

There are state and federal laws protecting you from being financially wiped out by the high cost of catastrophic illness. Many middle-income families do not realize that they do not have to sell their homes, bankrupt their future and go into debt forever. Your political representatives (local, state and federal) are aware of these laws and methods. Make them hear your plea for help. An attorney, paralegal, social services rep, or sometimes a knowledgeable librarian can help you locate the information you need to protect you from financial disaster. These protective laws have been written with just such emergencies in mind. Use them.

In many states, so long as you pay *something* (sometimes as little as a dollar) each month on your bill, you cannot be sued. Sometimes, so long as you pay taxes and interest on your property, it cannot be taken away from you.

If you are tired or confused or if you are emotionally drained and cannot deal intelligently with the financial situation in which you find yourself, ask a friend or family member removed from the problem and more knowledgeable, or an attorney or tax consultant to represent your cause in the problem areas.

Do not be intimidated or allow yourself to be forced into selling everything you own or into declaring bankruptcy. Do not become hysterical or defeated. You *can* come out of these difficulties with pride and property if you can keep calm and use the system instead of letting it abuse you.

Credit

If you don't have a credit rating, get one! In this age of plastic money it's difficult to find an adult who does not have a credit rating, but they do exist. If you are among this nearly extinct breed, it is imperative that you establish a credit record as quickly as possible. Why? Because like it or not, whether you approve of credit spending or not, you will need it sooner or later to purchase, to prove the checks you write are good or that you are financially responsible.

Generally speaking, you do not have a credit rating unless

120

you have borrowed money. However, you may share a credit rating with your spouse, in which case you would be advised only to check your credit rating through your bank or savings and loan. If you do not have a credit rating, it may be advisable for you to borrow, say $500 from your bank, deposit the money if you don't need it, and pay off the debt promptly out of the deposit funds, thus establishing credit at the cost of the interest being charged. In any case, when a person or family is facing a terminal illness and the complications it always presents, it is wise to know exactly where you stand financially. You may not need to borrow, but you never know.

Bank Accounts

If bank accounts (checking and savings) are not "joint" and the accounts are solely in the name of the deceased, the account becomes a part of the estate and cannot be touched until the estate is settled.

Accounts held in the names of two people payable to either go to the survivor upon death of one of the parties in most states. If, however, the account exceeds a certain stipulated amount (in some states), the bank is required to freeze even a joint account and notify the State Treasurer that it has this account. Bankers request that as soon as it is emotionally possible, the survivor come to the bank and change the name on the account. *Different states have different regulations; this is just one more reason why people should become familiar with their bank's policies.*

Taxes

Many states require a tax report be filed with the state after death, whether or not there is any estate. Your attorney or the State Treasurer will furnish you with the proper forms.

Debts

The executor or administrator should be given all debts of the deceased and *only* he or she should be responsible for clearing those debts while settling the estate. Check and see if outstand-

121

ing debts (cars, appliances, boats, RV's, mortgages, etc.) are covered through credit life insurance policies.

Safety Deposit Boxes

Like bank accounts, safety deposit boxes are subject to state and federal regulations. If a safety deposit box is held in joint ownership, the survivor may open the box. However, in some states, there must be a representative of the State Treasury present. This representative will take an inventory of the contents. The reasons for this are obvious (taxes, for instance), but the inconvenience is equally obvious if important papers (certificates, wills, insurance policies) are needed. Therefore, it is important to consider what is in the safety deposit box before the death of a mate or partner and make photocopies for ready reference.

If a safety deposit box is held solely by the deceased, it cannot be opened except by the administrator or executor of the estate. If the administrator or executor is not known, a bank or court official may open the box to search for a will. In either case, a state representative must be present. This procedure differs according to state laws but generally, a safety deposit box cannot be opened even by someone holding Power of Attorney after the death of the owner.

Living Trust

An alternative to a Letter of Intent (see Appendix I, page 171) is a Living Trust. This is not a substitute for a Will, but is a complement to one and is subtly different from a Letter of Intent and is the form used in some states. It is a good idea to have a Living Trust drawn up as closely to the writing of one's will as possible.

A Living Trust provides for the transfer of *personal* belongings at the time of death (personal property includes cash, jewelry, stock, bonds, but *not real estate*). These trusts can be revocable (the property remaining under your control) or irrevocable (you have no further control of your property).

The signer of a Living Trust (the trustor) must appoint a trustee (another person or organization such as a bank or trust company) to oversee the property and provisions. However, in a revocable trust, one can revoke (cancel) the trust if one so chooses. The advantage of this kind of trust is that the property passes immediately to the beneficiaries named in the trust, without going through probate court (a court of proceeding established to settle estates).

It would be wise to discuss the advantages and implications of a Living Trust, Letter of Intent or any other vehicle of dispersing of an estate with an attorney.

Letter of Intent

This is a letter which is *not* a Will, but eliminates uncertainty and confusion as to the wishes of the deceased. *This letter does not substitute for a Will and should not be placed in a safety deposit box.* It should be given to the executor of the estate, the next of kin, or a close, trusted friend.

The letter should include the following:

1. The location of the Will
2. Funeral or burial instructions
3. Location of all important documents
4. Location of safety deposit box and where the keys can be found
5. A list and location of insurance policies (name, number, amount and beneficiary), health, accident and burial policies
6. Pension or stock sharing plans
7. Bank accounts (checking and savings)
8. Stocks and bonds and where they are located
9. Real estate holdings
10. Major properties (personal and business)
11. Instruction and direction on business management
12. Names, addresses and telephone numbers of advisors such as lawyers, insurance agents, clergy, accountants, bankers
13. Names of close relatives and friends with addresses and telephone numbers

123

14. A list of how certain personal effects should be dispersed, to whom and by whom
15. Any other requests not included in a Will

Once all the Very Important Papers have been gathered together as suggested on page 105, a Letter of Intent becomes relatively simple. It is a sort of gathering up of loose ends and a chance to express personal desires and preferences that otherwise might go unheeded. It can be a very informal letter, or it can be structured by an attorney. In many cases, it is a simple dictated statement that certain people receive certain personal possessions or that the final disposition of one's body after death be taken care of in a specified manner. It is the sort of thing that solves the problems of who will receive father's watch or mother's wedding ring, which is often the cause of family problems after a Will has been read.

The Living Bank
(A Computerized Referral Donor Program)

As medical and surgical procedures progressed, there has been an increasing need for a center for organ transplantation, therapy, medical research, and anatomical studies. The Living Bank International, a non-profit service organization chartered in 1968, is headquartered in Houston, Texas, and is affiliated with the Texas Medical Center. The Living Bank provides donor registration forms and Uniform Donor Cards which are the only legal documents needed under the Uniform Anatomical Gift Act. It provides coordination and referrals of anatomical donations to appropriate medical facilities nearest the place of the donor's death. When notified, The Living Bank immediately contacts these facilities and cooperates with eye banks, kidney transplant centers, and similar facilities in the rapid transfer of organs to the banks for future use in saving lives or giving sight to the blind.

There is no conflict between local organ banks and The Living Bank since referrals are made to these banks by The Living Bank. So that there will be no misunderstandings or conflicts about transplantation and the donor's wish to give to The Living Bank, it is very important that these wishes be

124

made known to next of kin and all family members well before death.

The time element is vital in most transplants (kidneys must be received within minutes, eyes within six to eight hours, skin and bones within twelve to twenty-four hours) and it is important to have donor information in place at the time of death.

This is what happens when a donor dies and The Living Bank is notified:

1. A data sheet is completed with all the necessary information.
2. Where necessary, a medical examiner is contacted.
3. The eye bank, skin bank, and other appropriate transplant facilities closest to the donor are notified.
4. If the donor has indicated the choice for vital organ donation, and if the organs are medically acceptable and The Living Bank has been notified in time for retrieval, the nearest transplant group is notified and a medical team is immediately dispatched. If donated organs are not needed in the geographical area, The Living Bank ascertains the nearest waiting recipient and notifies the appropriate transplant center for retrieval.
5. If the body has been given for anatomical study or research, the nearest medical school is notified. If the school cannot use the body for any reason, another school is notified in the area. The family will be advised of all facets of this donation. In some instances there may be expenses such as transportation charges to be paid by the family. The choice of donation is left up to the family. Remains will be cremated or buried according to the wishes of the deceased, provided arrangements are made prior to the acceptance by a medical school.

Removal of organs or parts for transplantation does not disfigure the body in any way nor does it interfere with funeral or memorial arrangements. No additional expenses are involved because of donation.

Protestant, Catholic and Jewish leaders support the transplant program, believing that there is no greater gift than the gift of life. The donor program offers this opportunity to everyone, regardless of religion, race or economic status. See form in Appendix I. There is always a member of The Living Bank on call twenty-four hours a day. For further information, contact:

The Living Bank
PO Box 6725
Houston, Texas 77265
(713) 528-2971
U.S.A.: 1-800-528-2971

Living Will

At a time when life-sustaining equipment is readily available and the scientific, academic, legal and philosophic lines are being drawn, at a time when arguments for and against the prolongation of life versus the quality of life are being debated from federal and state capitals to the living rooms and classrooms of the country, getting actively involved in decisions about how far medicine should take life-sustaining measures can leave the family of the terminally ill between the proverbial rock and a hard place.

Bob and I signed a Living Will long before such matters were openly discussed. We felt that quality of life was the most important factor. Our joint decision was based on philosophic, religious, and economic concerns.

After having periodically updated the Living Will over twenty years to comply with the statute of limitations, we found that previous photocopies of our decisions had been lost in the shuffle of medical records and so once again we had to emphasize to Bob's doctors that this was no passing fancy and it must be incorporated prominently in their files.

Oregon, where I live, has passed a Natural Death Act. In addition to the Living Will Bob and I prepared, there was a Directive to Physicians which I photocopied and gave to my

126

sons, my attorney, and my doctor. Since each state differs in regulations and opinions, it is important that you understand the laws governing your state. Information is readily available by writing to:

The Society for the Right to Die
250 West 57th Street
New York, New York 10107
(212) 246-6973

If you live in Alabama, Arkansas, California, Idaho, Kansas, Nevada, New Mexico, North Carolina, Oregon, Texas, Vermont, Washington or the District of Columbia, where right-to-die laws are on the books, The Society for the Right to Die will send you documents and guidelines along with the Living Will forms. The Living Will is respected by many doctors and hospitals where the right-to-die laws have not been legislated as yet. See sample form in Appendix I, p. 170. You can receive the information you need for your situation by contacting the Society. These important documents and guidelines benefit the patient, physician and hospital by clarifying the desires of a terminal patient.

Still another form which should be presented and enforced early on in a terminal illness is a Medical Power of Attorney (or Limited Power of Attorney), which gives the next of kin or designated person the right to make decisions in certain areas which the person who is ill may not be capable of making. Again, it is wise and important that this form be checked for legality in the place in which you live. Any attorney can help you with proper wording and the notarization of this form.

When you have presented photocopies of these documents to your physician and asked that they be included on both the hospital records and the physician's records, you have provided the best and only insurance against artificial prolongation of life.

There is a third request that can be made by or for the terminally ill patient who wishes to be allowed to die without extreme or heroic measures. It is a written request that there be a "No Code" statement attached to his hospital records by

127

the attending physician. This statement is to tell care-givers that if vital signs are diminishing or have ceased, no extreme measures other than those which will bring comfort to a patient should be administered.

Each of these decisions and forms should be carefully considered and agreed upon as soon as possible—even before illness is an issue—so that your wishes and the desires of the person who is dying are clearly stated and clearly understood by those who direct the care of a patient.

This is not euthanasia—it is a simple request not to be artificially sustained when death would be the natural outcome of the illness. Should your doctor not agree (and there are some who will not), there will be other doctors equally capable who will accept the decision of a rational person that he or she be allowed to die with dignity and as naturally as possible.

Death Benefits

Social Security Death Benefits
Because Social Security benefits are changing in both amount and method of distribution, exact requirements are difficult to spell out. The best way to get current information is to contact the nearest Social Security office. However, there are certain documents you will need in order to prove eligibility. These include the following:

1. Social Security card number.
2. A record of earnings for the year prior to death or disability.
3. Certified birth certificates for spouse and all children under eighteen years of age.
4. Death certificate.

Benefits may include either a lump sum death payment or a survivor's monthly benefit for those eligible (at this writing that includes minors, dependent spouses over 60 years of age, disabled spouses, and dependent parents over age 62).

There are time limitations and other regulations involved in Social Security benefits and so it is important to go to a

Social Security office as soon as possible if you think you are eligible.

Veteran's Benefits

At this writing families of veterans with honorable discharges or general discharges under honorable conditions are eligible for death benefits. Your funeral director or your attorney will be able to guide you in applying for veteran's benefits. In most county courthouses there are representative officers who can give you details about possible state and federal benefits. Take the veteran's discharge papers and a certified copy of the death certificate with you when you go to the Veterans' Administration Office or the local Veterans' Officer.

Possible benefits include pensions to the surviving spouse, aid and attendance benefits, educational aid for a spouse and/or children, burial allowance, burial in a national cemetery, burial flag, headstone or grave marker, G.I. insurance, tax exemptions in some states, employment assistance for survivors, free copies of military, marriage, divorce, death and birth records when needed to support claims.

Possible Employee Benefits

A survivor or your attorney should check with the deceased's employer for any benefits due the family. Under employment contracts there may be pensions or profit-sharing plans, annuities, death benefits, unpaid wages or salary, widow's pensions, group insurance, and employee medical, health and hospitalization plans. In the case of accidental or industrial-related death, there may be insurance policies giving additional benefits. Give all employee policies to your attorney so that he can help you understand and make proper claims.

Life Insurance

The company agent of the deceased's life insurance policy will assist you at no cost for his/her services in signing claims. There are usually five options open to you at this time:

1. *Lump Sum.* Taking the entire face value of the policy.

2. *Interest Option.* Money is left with the insurance company and will collect interest until needed.
3. *Time Option.* An option that pays monthly payments over an allotted period of time designated by beneficiary.
4. *Amount Option.* A regular income of as much money as the beneficiary requires for as long as money and interest last.
5. *Lifetime Income Option.* A regular income option.

Before making a decision it is wise to discuss these alternatives with an attorney, banker, or financial advisor who has the expertise to guide you through the decision-making process. Check to see if the deceased was covered by life insurance in his work, fraternal organization or some other group. Check to see if the deceased had *credit-life insurance* on any outstanding debts (automobile, home, appliances, boat, etc.).

CHAPTER · *13*

Memorial and Funeral Planning

Along with gentle birthing, personal marriage vows and death with dignity has come the encouragement and acceptance of individual funeral or memorial services. More and more people recognize the right and need to plan their final rites and it has become possible to plan the service you want for yourself or a loved one without fear of social stigma.

Arranging a funeral is a thing most people postpone until something or someone forces the issue. If, however, each of us set aside one hour to briefly state on paper what our wishes are as to the disposition of our remains, the kind of memorial service we desire, and our favorite music, scripture, prose or poetry, we would remove much of the anguish families must deal with at a time when they are least able to cope.

The death of a loved one is an emotional experience, and to avoid mistakes in judgment it's necessary to be objective and knowledgeable about what can be expected from the time of death until the final disposition of the body. Planning simplifies this confusing time and clarifies the desires of the deceased. See Letter of Intent, Appendix I, page 171. Preparing for a funeral allows a person to compare costs and make sound judgments as to what they *really* want and how much it will cost. It does not necessitate prepayment or financing. It simply gives a funeral director necessary information to serve you best. When death occurs, a telephone call is all you need to carry out the loved one's desires, which were made when they were able to think clearly.

Costs will vary and will depend on the number of services rendered. Generally speaking, however, there are four separate charges for a funeral. If you are familiar with these charges before they are needed, you will be better prepared, financially and emotionally, to deal with them. It is important to find out from your funeral director *exactly* which of his services are included as *professional services* and which are *optional services*, which involve additional charges.

Professional funeral services generally include embalming, cosmetology, arrangements for a memorial or religious service, preparation of government certificates, notification of pall bearers, arrangement for handling flowers or donations, eulogy (memorial) cards, use of staff facilities and basic transportation. Often these services are categorized so that if one or more of the above items are to be deleted, the cost is lowered.

Optional funeral service expenses, if provided by the director, may include flowers, burial clothing, limousines (in addition to basic transportation), music, death or funeral notices, transportation of the body for cremation or distant burial, long distance telephone calls or telegrams. Many state laws require the funeral director to provide a cost list of all services provided. Be sure to request that the cost of any service be documented and signed *before* the director is hired and any agreement is reached.

Caskets are a costly item. Prices range from $100 or $200 to $1,500 and upwards. Choosing a suitable coffin within an affordable price range ought to be carefully considered—one reason why prearrangement is so important. It is possible to purchase a fiberboard container for cremation which lowers the cost of a funeral by thousands of dollars.

Embalming and cosmetology is generally not required by law if the body is buried or cremated within 24 hours after death. If it is to be held longer than that, it must be embalmed or refrigerated. Embalming is required as a health measure, and cosmetology is a separate procedure used to restore the features of the deceased to his/her former likeness. The funeral director can explain these options and the legal requirements of the law where you live.

Arrangements for a memorial or religious service is a personal option. More and more frequently family and friends choose a service which reflects the personality, philosophy, life and values of the person who died. The funeral director is trained to help you choose a service appropriate to your needs and desires. If you don't have a minister, priest or rabbi, the director will put you in touch with one and you can relay the information about the deceased, giving a personalized touch to the service. If you have a religious counselor, let him/her guide you in the choice of a funeral service. The honorarium given to the clergy for his/her services depends on your generosity and financial circumstances. The funeral director can tell you the appropriate or customary amount in your area.

Cemeteries—interment receptacles, cemetery lots and disposition of remains—all require clear, level-headed decisions and should never be made when one is under emotional stress. Before you commit yourself to any decisions regarding cemeteries, burial lots, or interment receptacles, bring along a level-headed member of your family, a friend, or a trusted adviser to give you the perspective and advice you need. Cemeteries often require that caskets be placed in an *interment receptacle* to reduce possible grave cave-ins or disturbances. These receptacles can be made of concrete, steel, copper or fiberglass. They are purchased through the funeral director or cemetery. The cost varies but, generally nationwide, concrete or fiberglass are the least expensive.

Cemetery service charges are separate charges from those made for caskets, services and receptacles. They include the opening and closing of the grave and the interment and recording fees. Usually this cost is covered by the person who is making the funeral arrangements, but in some cases, the funeral director includes these costs in funeral arrangements and will expect reimbursement. *Again, get the funeral director's services and costs before you sign an agreement.*

133

Cemetery lots will vary in cost depending on location, maintenance and, in some cases, ownership (privately owned, church- or lodge-owned or national). Some people have family plots, in which case planning has been taken care of. Veterans have the right to be buried in a national cemetery depending on available space, and the surviving spouse and children are allowed by law to be buried at the same grave site. These arrangements are made by reservation; funeral directors have all the information you will need.

A good rule of thumb to remember when considering a cemetery lot is that there are national organizations that maintain high standards among their members, and there are state organizations which try to keep standards and practices high and honorable. Check credentials through the Better Business Bureau or a reputable funeral director.*

When choosing a cemetery lot, there are six points one should carefully consider:

1. Choose a lot in a cemetery managed by reputable people. Avoid places where there are high-pressure sales or where "bargain" and "give-away" schemes are offered. If you have any doubts, ask your clergy, or check with the BBB or Funeral Director's Association.
2. Have "perpetual care" or "endowed care" spelled out in *writing* and check to see if the endorsed-care funds are carefully guarded (invested) and that there are adequate reserve funds available for maintenance.
3. Know *exactly* where the lot is located and check the location personally. *Never* depend on maps or drawings provided by salesmen or owners.
4. Compare prices with other lots in the cemetery and with other cemeteries in the community.
5. Check the kinds and prices of monuments and markers within the cemetery to see if they are pleasing to you. Find out the policy of grave decoration to see if it fits your needs or offends you.

* *See names and addresses at end of chapter.*

134

6. Get the price of grave opening and closing and the cost of setting grave markers or monuments *in writing.* (Sometimes the cemetery lot costs are low but the other costs extremely high.)

If the plan for burial is on *private property* and is permissible under the laws of your state, local health officials and other appropriate state or county agencies will have to be notified. The funeral director will have the information you will need under the circumstances.

Mausoleums usually contain a series of vaults for entombment. Many cemeteries have mausoleums on their grounds and you will need the same information in considering mausoleums as in choosing a cemetery lot. Opening and closing a crypt involves costs which should be clearly spelled out *in writing.*

In these days of mobility, it is quite possible the family may choose to ship the body to another part of the country for burial. Despite beliefs to the contrary, it is not required by law that anyone accompany the body. Commercial airlines provide this service and a funeral director will have all the necessary information.

Cremation is another option in the disposition of remains. As in any other funeral service, a container or casket is used. Often a fiberboard container is chosen, which considerably lowers the cost of a more elaborate casket. The number of professional services and supplemental services will affect the total cost of the funeral, and since cremation often necessitates transporting the body from the funeral parlor to a crematorium, it may be important to find out the cost, and if an equally satisfactory funeral home with a crematory is conveniently located.

Often in the case of cremation, a memorial service without the body present is preferred. If this is the case, the family will have several options for dealing with the remains.

The cremated remains may be placed in a container. The family may opt for providing an urn of their choice. Urn prices can range from $35–$50 to thousands of dollars. Urns

135

can be placed in a mausoleum, buried in a cemetery, kept at home or in a *columbarium*, which is a special edifice in a cemetery. The funeral director can provide you with the options and the cost. Scattering of cremated remains is another option. If this is to be done, ask the funeral director for the legalities in the area you have chosen.

Monuments and/or markers need not be chosen at the time you arrange for funeral services and disposition of remains. You should, however, find out any restrictions on size or placement when you make arrangements with the cemetery.

Be sure to shop around for the grave marker. You have the time, since it need not be decided at once, to compare for quality, workmanship, and cost and to make your decision when you are more rested and able to cope.

Notices are customarily placed in the death, funeral and obituary sections of newspapers. At the request of the family, the funeral director will take care of these notices and will charge the family for this service. By collecting vital information as suggested on page 108, you can assist the funeral director more easily in providing important information in the obituary.

An *autopsy* is sometimes requested by the attending physician. Under the law, the family may give or deny permission, unless the deceased has died under violent or suspicious circumstances. An autopsy, for whatever reason, does not disfigure the body or delay funeral services.

The *donation of organs* or the body is covered in detail on page 124, "The Living Bank." Your attending physician or funeral director should know your intention regarding organ or body donation.

The following checklist will be helpful if it's readily available at the time of death, and copies should be given to those who will be involved in the funeral arrangements and services:

1. Funeral home—location and telephone number.
2. Disposition of remains—burial/cremation/crypt/ mausoleums.

3. Clergy—name and telephone number.
4. Burial clothing—brief description and location.
5. Music—who is in charge, special requests, telephone numbers.
6. Family and friends to be notified—names and numbers.
7. Flowers/Cards/ Acknowledgments—who will be in charge?
8. Fraternal and professional organizations to be notified—who will be in charge? Names and telephone numbers.
9. Pallbearers—names, addresses and telephone numbers.
10. Out-of-town accommodations—who will be in charge? Names and telephone numbers.
11. Letter of Intent and Will—location, name and telephone number of executor, name and telephone number of attorney.
12. Host or hostess to be in charge of refreshments and other religious customs of predeath and afterdeath gatherings and services.
13. Transportation assistance—who will meet out-of-town friends and relations? Names and telephone numbers.
14. Photocopies of Very Important Papers (see Legalities and Decisions section, pages 109–12)—location of these documents.

These fourteen suggestions will take a great deal of pressure off a grieving family and allow for the healing process to take place. It is a kindness to allow others who have cared about your loved one to share these final rites. If you ask in advance of death, friends and family members will have time to organize and do their best in helping this final tribute go smoothly.

Further information may be obtained from:
Continental Associations of Funeral & Memorial Societies
50 E. Van Buren St.
Chicago, Ill.   60605

The American Way of Death by Jessica Mitford also has a list of memorial societies.

The International Order of the Golden Rule
P.O. Box 3586
Springfield, Ill.   62708
National Funeral Director's Association
(See local directory)

PART FOUR

Special Considerations

CHAPTER · 14

Making Visiting Easier

Any sensitive person finds it difficult and depressing to visit the terminally ill. Facing a loved one in the final stage of life can be quite unsettling, but faithfulness is the badge of love and dodging your responsibilities can lead to emotional and spiritual dilemmas later on.

The last few months of life naturally become a time of privacy and introspection, and we should not intrude or force a patient to extend energy beyond his/her tolerance. There are many ways we can bring the warmth, comfort and companionship that lessens the isolation and rejection many dying persons feel.

Instead of making up lame excuses ("He probably won't recognize me"; "I'd be intruding"; "I don't know how to act or what to say . . . "; "I'll cry or fall apart if I see him/her suffering"), we can arm ourselves with a few sound guidelines and spare ourselves the guilt and embarrassment of hurting people we love by ignoring them at the time of greatest need.

When a person is ill and at home, *call ahead* and ask when the best visiting time is, and if there is anything about the patient's condition you should be aware of (changes in hearing, sight, behavior). Also, ask if there is anything you can bring to the patient or care-giver.

Often a newly released hospital patient is depressed— environment changes of any kind can deplete energy. Every aspect of the patient's life is changed in this instance and it may take as long as a week for your loved one to adjust. Your visit and understanding can bring stability and continuity to the patient. You are familiar and beloved. You represent happier times when vigor and control were an ordinary part of living. So accept any depression or confusion and simply try to understand the patient's suffering. Your visit will be a success.

Time yourself based on the care-giver's recommendation, who knows best the patient's strength and capacity. Five to fifteen minutes is adequate and considerate when a person is gravely ill. Prolonged visits will defeat the purpose of your visit. Patients will tell you that the concept of time in a sickroom is different from time anywhere else. Medication, drugs and pain put a person in a time-warp that speeds and/or creeps according to conditions. When you arrive, state that you will be there for a few minutes. Leave before fatigue sets in and you will be doing everyone concerned with this patient a great kindness.

Many people make the mistake of visiting a sick person with mutual friends. This may bolster the courage of the visitor but it cheats the person you are visiting of private, quality time with you. Just as too many cooks spoil the broth, too many visitors spoil the visit. It is a trial rather than a pleasure for a sick person to try to follow a conversation with more than one person, especially when under medication or in pain.

Make your visit one that focuses totally on the patient. Give him/her your undivided attention and let him/her lead the conversation. Time is short for the two of you to share whatever has bound you in love and friendship before this illness. But if he or she has a television going or seems reluctant to talk, share the time by accepting the conditions set before you. Nonverbal communication can sometimes be as satisfactory as talking. What's crucial is that *you are there*.

What can you *bring* to a dying patient? Mostly you will bring love, but if you bring a gift, make it one that can easily be cared for in the sickroom. The following gifts were most popular with patients in hospitals, convalescent homes, and at home:

- Cosmetics: Light, fragrant powder, cologne, body lotion, after-shave lotion, soap, etc.
- Cassettes: Favorite music, poetry, scriptural readings, etc. You can tape them at home and personalize them
- A soft cardigan or bed jacket with long, loose sleeves to protect arms and elbows from linen burns (sheets sometimes cause uncomfortable rashes)
- A colorful afghan or lightweight lap robe
- A selection of mints, lifesavers, breath fresheners, lemon drops, etc.
- Note paper, pen, stamps, notebook, etc.
- A snapshot or poster of a beloved place or pet to tape on the wall
- Homemade soup, cookies, or snacks in disposable containers
- A package of special tea bags or packets of instant soups or coffee
- A bottle of wine or brandy (if permitted by the doctor)
- A gift certificate for a massage, shampoo, manicure, pedicure, etc.
- A balloon bouquet or balloon message (unless the patient hallucinates)
- Large-print magazines or newspapers or picture magazines for the sight-impaired
- Sample-sized mouthwashes, shampoos, lotions, etc.
- A small stuffed animal
- An ant farm or terrarium if they are allowed
- A basket assortment of small wrapped gifts—one for each day until you come back

What do you say to a person who is dying? Naturally, it will depend on the condition, personality, receptiveness, and your relationship, but the best rule to follow is to let the patient set not only the tone and pace, but the topics of conversation. Here are some guidelines:

- Reminisce if it's appropriate. Refresh yourself and him/her with the good things you have shared.
- Don't try to divert the friend from a topic he/she wants to discuss.

143

- Don't be afraid to discuss death—let your beloved one express deep feelings. Don't lie, even politely. Be evasive, be diplomatic; but don't lie.
- Let him/her cry. Fear of sharing the grief of parting is probably the deepest fear you both are feeling. Expressing those feelings of fear and grief is natural during some phases of a terminal illness. If the *patient* initiates tears and expresses that grief, share it.
- Let the patient talk, even if it's repetitious. Keep quiet and let the person express him/herself. A sympathetic listener is far more important than a brilliant conversationalist just now.
- Reassure—don't argue or explain how you feel. Let it be known that, despite any guilty feelings either one of you may have over the past and what has happened, you think he/she is special and good and worthy.
- Weep if it's natural, share hurts and sorrows. *Don't* tell a dying person to "buck up" or be brave.
- Touch—a hand being held, a brow being kissed, or a hug is important. Don't be afraid of contact and affection. They are more necessary than medicine now.
- *Ask* what you can do and do it. Keep your promises.
- If your loved one cannot converse, be quiet and just be there. Don't talk over or around the patient—he/she is the focal point of this visit. Talk to care-givers and others *away* from the patient. (You wouldn't exclude this person from conversations if he/she were well—don't do it now.)
- Find out if there is a need to talk about his/her condition. Do it by simply asking, "Do you want to talk about it?"
- Offer to answer correspondence, shop or do errands, call mutual friends, etc.
- Be prepared for the patient's anger, depression or a "high." Don't take barbs or sarcasm personally. Feel flattered that you are close enough and dear enough to risk the sharing of fears, angers, denials, or frustrations.

144

- Discuss only the news that's important *to him or her.* Don't prattle.
- Don't lecture or preach. Whatever caused the illness is not your business. Support, sympathize, and *love.* Period!
- If you are aware there are certain conversational irritations that patients complain about, you can avoid them. On the surface they seem trivial, but they become profound, especially during a prolonged illness. When interviewing dying patients I heard quite a few complaints. Number one was being asked, "How are you?" It's such a common greeting we don't realize the impact it may have on a dying person. One patient retaliated by answering, "I'm dying, thank you, how are you?" Another said he answered by saying "How the hell do you think I'm feeling?" Most patients felt that a simple "Hello" or perhaps "I'm glad to see you" was sufficient.

Hovering around a person who is dying distresses many of them. If you can be there when and as needed without making them feel you are fearful and constantly on the alert to every breath or spasm, sick people feel more comfortable. Allow the patients to ask for assistance. It gives them a feeling of some control.

Watch your tone of voice when conversing with a patient. Don't shout; speak clearly and enunciate your words. A feisty little lady stated, "I may be dying but, by golly, my ears still work!" It irritates patients to hear someone say, "It's time for *our* shot or *our* medicine or *our* bath or *our* dinner" and drives them bananas to be talked to like a child. Most resent cutesy baby talk, and all seemed to hate condescension.

- Remember the good times. Isn't this a time when remembering can bring a smile, a laugh, and a warm glow that will last after you are gone?
- If he/she is ambulatory, perhaps a ride or visit to a favorite place can be arranged. Remember physical limitations and secure a physician's permission and approval.

- Celebrate holidays by dropping in for a minute, calling to say you remember, or sending a shower of cards. A room decoration appropriate to the holiday is always welcome. Talk about past shared holidays.

Hope is important; miracles happen. Hope with him or her and don't clam up when the future is mentioned. Sometimes hope is all a person has to cling to. When one is facing the greatest unknown, hope should not be denied. Share it, give it, trust in it. Remember, "Perfect love believes all things, *hopes* all things, endures all things." (New Testament)

If the patient has entered a world beyond your understanding, if the mind wanders or if the patient no longer can or will talk, don't run away. Sit quietly, hold a hand if it's appropriate—and grow. You are witnessing the mystical withdrawal from life seldom seen in today's run-and-hide society. Chances are your loved one will sense your presence and *you* will respond to that unspoken connection. This moment—I promise—will be a blessing and a holy memory when the pain has passed.

Be grateful for the remaining time left for you and your loved one and let the patient know how glad you are that you shared life with him or her. Don't allow your discomfort at intimacy to rob you of the obligation and pleasure of saying thank you.

Remember, if you can, that many people withdraw from death because of fear, frustration and helplessness. If your visit can make this particular time, day or week, more comfortable and a little happier for a loved one, you will have given the most precious gift of all—*love.*

CHAPTER · *15*

Nontraditional Couples

All nontraditional couples, whatever their commitment to one another, face common problems. They have property combinations (who originally owned what, etc.), financial arrangements (household expenses, joint ownership), past relationships to be considered (families and friends), and professional considerations. Ideally these problems should be resolved prior to any crisis, but often they lie unsolved until there is a crisis.

Illness and death can do strange things to the reasoning of otherwise dependable people. Property ownership and legal rights are at best a sensitive area, but in a crisis situation, where nontraditional couples have jointly accrued and pooled their resources, being legally unprepared can be not only heartbreaking but unbelievably exhausting under most of our present state laws.

When two consenting adults choose to live together they are entering a fragile and precarious legal relationship. The sooner ownership and disposition of property is discussed and legally clarified, the better are the chances that the intentions of both partners are apt to stand up in a court of law if and when there comes a time of determination.

The samples of various legal forms in Appendix I can serve as guides to help you protect your partner, and the lists of important documents you may need should be readily available.

People often make the mistake of believing that spelling out their wishes in their will (for instance, to be cremated or buried in a certain place), will guarantee those things will happen. Not so! The time between death and the reading of a will is a critical period when donation of organs and disposition of remains will be made. (See Letter of Intent.)

Since you are not considered next of kin, in most current couple relationships, you should be aware that many states require the next of kin to sign documentation for organ donation and cremation, etc., regardless of the written directions given by the deceased. When a partner is terminally ill it is terribly important that an attorney be contacted as soon as possible to the time of diagnosis and the partners' wishes be made known. A legally sound document will save painful conflicts in the future.

In every city of any size there will be legal advice available. The gay and lesbian communities in these cities can put you in touch with attorneys who are legally prepared for those living in a nontraditional partnership. Of course, all nontraditional couples can be advised through the Legal Aid Society as to how to meet their needs.

Lesbians and gays living a nontraditional lifestyle find that the many problems of stress and grief during terminal illness are more complicated for them than for those living in the straight community. Sometimes these complications are due to the oppression many experience, but often the problems lie in their own passivity in dealing with areas of legal rights, social services, and spiritual needs.

At a time when you are overburdened by stress, conflicts and emotions, finding the necessary help to carry you through the crisis of dying and death of your partner is critical. If the "traditional" community withdraws the spiritual and emotional support you need, you must find someone—*anyone*—who will do the necessary legwork and research within the nontraditional community for the kind of help you need.

After spending months trying to track down a central clearing house where gay couples can get information and support for medical, legal and emotional needs, I found ample and growing support nationwide for AIDS patients and their loved ones built on a growing awareness of the needs of those who suffer from other terminal illnesses.

Legal assistance *is* available for those who take the initiative to contact Gay Rights organizations.* There *are* ministers, priests, and rabbis; doctors, psychologists, social workers, and activists sympathetic and willing to help. If you are too weary or confused to seek help personally, again, find a friend who will do the calling and letter writing necessary to let your needs be known. There is a list of organizations and associations listed under "Support, Information and Referrals," (p. 182).

If there is a Shanti (hospice for AIDS victims) nearby, contact them. Often Shanti can match their carefully selected and trained personnel to meet the needs of people facing life-threatening problems on a confidential basis.

Essentially, it is up to the nontraditional couples to put aside hangups and rally to the needs of one another, and to take an active role in seeking the help that is readily available to those who seek it.

Family problems—the acceptance or rejection of a person's partner by parents, ex-spouses, and children—is often a problem in nontraditional relationships. Often it takes a third party trained in human relations—someone with an understanding heart—to heal the rift that comes with the decision to choose an alternative lifestyle. If anger, guilt, pride, etc., prevent healing the breach in a relationship, find that third person—clergy, social worker, mutual friend, understanding family member. The past cannot be changed but the present and the future can be made more tenable by accepting and remembering the good things that happen in all relationships and putting aside the bitterness.

When time is short, time is precious. Living in harmony is always better than living in discord—and so it is with dying. Now is the time to remember that love is not sitting in judgment; it is trusting and accepting.

* See Gay Rights National Lobby,
P. O. Box 1892
Washington, D.C.

What to Do When a Friend Has AIDS

The shadow cast by AIDS darkens even as education of the homosexual community and society in general is accelerated. Rather than go into often-repeated assurances that AIDS cannot be communicated except by sexual contact, IV drug users, contacts with prostitutes, and (prior to screening procedures) through blood products, this section deals only with suggestions offered by Shanti, GMHC, *Make Today Count*, and hospice organizations which have been dealing longest with AIDS victims and those close to them:

1. Call before you plan to visit because he may not feel strong enough to have a visitor today. If he can't see you immediately, call back until you find a day when you'll be welcome—or tell him to call you when he's up to seeing you.

2. Help his lover, care-partner, or roommate, who is also suffering fatigue, fear and grief. Offer to spend the afternoon—or a weekend—to give loved ones a break. Or invite the care-giver to dinner or a show to give him a change of pace and change of scenery.

3. If the patient is a parent, ask what you can do for the children. Take them on an outing or to visit their parent.

4. Allow him the right to make decisions; allow him to be as independent as possible.

5. If transportation is needed to see the doctor, therapist, the bank, grocery store or any other place, offer to take him.

6. Don't allow the patient or the care-giver to feel isolated. Get in touch with support groups and old friends who want to help. If there is no support group in your community, organize one.

7. Don't allow the patient to blame himself for contracting AIDS. It's *not his fault*.

8. If you are going to be intimate, be absolutely certain you understand all the precautions *both* of you should take.

9. Allow the patient and his partner to hope and genuinely hope with them. Hope may be the ingredient that will keep him alive until there is a medical breakthrough.
10. If depressed, angry or noncommunicative, accept these moods. A true friend can share even the bad moods.
11. Don't be afraid to touch. You cannot contact AIDS by holding a hand or hugging.
12. Food prepared and brought in disposable containers is most welcome to both partners in an AIDS household. Perhaps you could organize a group of friends to prepare a meal once or twice a week. It would be a wonderful change.

People with AIDS and their loved ones are caught in a double bind. There is the debilitating illness itself and the hysteria of society in general. Take the disease seriously, but remember that it's the isolation and homophobia that hurt as badly as the disease. Sometimes a gay man has only his gay friends and lover(s) as family. Be a loving family member, apply the Golden Rule and bring warmth and love to these last days.

Whom to Contact for AIDS Assistance
Resource information and assistance are available if you persevere. The GMHC* and other gay and lesbian organizations are invaluable sources because they have a national network and organized support groups within the gay community. GMHC has an 800 number to answer questions and offer help immediately.

Be prepared for crisis by checking out the availability of homecare attendants, financial aid counselors, therapists, recreational groups, and self-help demonstrators who can teach relaxation therapy, visual imagery, touch communication, etc.

* All addresses and 800 numbers are listed in Appendix II "Support, Information and Referral Sources."

151

If you can make it your responsibility to learn *ahead* of time of crisis (a crisis as defined by GMHC is *a serious or decisive state—a turning point*) what to do and where to find assistance, you will have removed much of the stress, exhaustion and turmoil to which many patients with AIDS and their partners have been subjected.

It is important that you keep *current* on information and support assistance through agencies such as GMHC and/or the National Gay Task force, U.S. Department of Health and Human Services and other organizations listed in Appendix II.

AIDS is a new life-threatening disease—it is not a death warrant. It arrived suddenly (1979–80) and the incidents of the disease grew rapidly. But the best-informed researchers feel that it will soon be controlled and will diminish as a threat as suddenly as polio and diptheria. Meanwhile, new and positive developments are discovered every day. Greater support is now being offered to AIDS patients by the heterosexual and religious communities which have often been hostile, judgmental and homophobic.

It is to your advantage and the advantage of your loved one that you make it a point to know the latest medical, therapeutic and social resources and accept the guidance of those who have our well-being uppermost in mind and heart.

Note: The information, guidance and Buddy Training Manual offered by GMHC should be within easy reach to everyone concerned with AIDS whether one is actively involved in the problems and prevention or is simply an interested bystander.

152

CHAPTER 16

Care of the Elderly

BEATITUDES FOR AGING

Blessed are they who understand
My faltering steps and palsied hand
Blessed are they who know my ears today
Must strain to catch the words they say
Blessed are they who seem to know that my eyes
Are dim and my wits are slow.
Blessed are they who look away when coffee
Spilled on the table today
Blessed are they with a cherry smile who stop to
Chat for a little while.
Blessed are they who never say, "You've told that story
twice today."
Blessed are they who know the ways to bring back
Memories of yesterdays
Blessed are they who make it known
That I'm loved, respected and not alone.
Blessed are they who know I'm at a loss
To find the strength to carry my cross
Blessed are they who ease the days
On my journey Home in loving ways.

*—**Author unknown***

The care of the elderly sick and dying is one of the principal problems facing American families today. Until recently, the care of an elderly family member was considered the duty, responsibility and normal inevitability for American families. When there was no Social Security and other insurance programs, there was no doubt as to who would take over the care of the old ones. "Putting away" an elderly relative was considered contemptible and abusive and was not an economically feasible answer to the problem.

The social reforms that followed World War II changed all that. Smaller homes excluded the possibility of additional family members. Children moving greater distances from parents sometimes alienated the young from the old. Two-paycheck families left no one at home to carry out domestic and nursing duties. Increasingly unable to communicate with others, people began to experience subtle changes in values and question their traditional responsibilities. One such area of change was the attitude of children toward their aging parents.

When Social Security and Medicare became available to the elderly, options for care seemed to narrow; that is, in order to receive financial help for the ridiculously high-cost care often needed by the elderly, older patients must be placed in facilities approved by the bureaucracy and thus, fired by government subsidies, the costs continued upward and the problem of care for the elderly multiplied—and continue to escalate.

There are no easy answers to the often lengthy and debilitating illness preceding the closing weeks or months of life. However, when the terminal patient is elderly, brain-impaired, heavily medicated or emotionally depressed, it is *imperative* that the person responsible for the kind of care he receives in his last days be aware of patient's rights in a skilled, professional nursing facility or any out-of-home care location.

Every state handles rules and regulations governing these facilities and a call or note to the Legal Aid Society nearest you will provide you with the information you need as to how your state enforces patient's rights. If these rights and regulations are not in effect, an attorney can insist that important stipulations be a part of the contract the patient and/or his family sign when entering the facility.

The State of California Skilled Nursing Facilities Regulation (Section 72523) is generally considered at this writing to be an acceptable model by which to judge the competency,

154

quality of care, and level of concern for patients in such facilities. Every patient admitted to facilities adhering to these regulations has these rights:

1. To be fully informed of his rights of all rules and regulations of the nursing home governing patient conduct.
2. To be fully informed of the services available in the facility and the cost of those services.
3. To be fully informed by a physician of his medical condition (except where limited by a physician and where medically inadvisable); to have the opportunity to participate in the planning of his medical treatment and to refuse to participate in medical research.
4. To refuse treatment to the extent permitted by law and to be informed of the medical consequences of refusal.
5. To be transferred or discharged only for medical reasons, or for his welfare or that of other patients, or for nonpayment for his stay—and to be given reasonable advance notice.
6. To be encouraged and assisted throughout his period of stay to exercise his rights as a patient and as a citizen—free from restraint, interference, coercion, discrimination or reprisal.
7. To manage his personal financial affairs, or to be given, at least quarterly, an accounting of financial transactions made on his behalf if the facility accepts this responsibility for him.
8. To be free from mental or physical abuse and from chemical and (except in emergencies) physical restraints except as authorized in writing by a physician for a specified and limited period of time, or, when necessary, to protect the patient from injury to himself or to others.
9. To be assured confidential treatment of his personal and medical records.
10. To be treated with consideration, respect and full

recognition of his dignity and individuality, including privacy in treatment and in care for his personal needs.

11. Not to be required to perform services for the facility that are not included in his plan of care for therapeutic purposes.

12. To associate and communicate privately with persons of his choice, and to send and receive his personal mail unopened, except where this right may be limited by a physician and is not medically advisable.

13. To meet with and participate in activities of social, religious, and community groups at his discretion, except where limited by his physician as a medical necessity.

14. To retain and use his personal clothing and possessions as space permits unless it would infringe on the rights of other patients.

15. If married, to be assured privacy for visits by his/her spouse; if both are patients in the facility, to be permitted to share a room (unless medically inadvisable).

16. To have daily visiting hours established.

17. To have members of the clergy admitted at the request of the patient or person responsible for the patient at any time.

18. To allow relatives or persons responsible to visit critically ill patients at any time (unless limited by the patient's physician for medical reasons).

19. To be allowed privacy for visits for professional or business purposes as well as visits from family, friends, clergy, or social workers.

20. To have reasonable access to telephones both to make and receive confidential calls.

These 20 points were excerpted from the California Department of Justice Information Pamphlet #7, *Understanding the New California Nursing Home Law*, Euell J. Younger, Attorney General, 1978.

Regardless of the state of mind and/or body, no person should be placed in a nursing facility which refuses to adhere to the rights outlined above. It is incumbent upon whomever is legally in charge or morally obligated in the care of the elderly to check *each and every* facet of care.

There may be times when caring for the elderly at home becomes impossible. The guilt engendered by horror stories of neglect in nursing homes has made the decision to place the elderly in a nursing facility a nightmare for concerned families. In addition to the California regulations in this section, please refer to the chapter "Convalescent/ Nursing Homes," for additional guidance in the physical care of the elderly.

But what of the less tangible provisions for an aged patient? Only *you* can provide the attention and tenderness needed to sustain an older person isolated from the people and places he/she loves. Often it is not pain or disease that breaks a spirit, but the loneliness of wondering *why* life has become so desolate.

An elderly cancer patient I visited said, "Be sure to tell people we miss touching. You can't know how awful it is to never be hugged or kissed by someone you love. I think they bring kittens and dogs in to see us because *they* like to be petted. Kittens and dogs and children aren't scared of us." I left with a lump in my throat wishing I could send a hug a day into that ward.

Go often to see your elderly patient. Even if you are not recognized, your love will be felt. Your name may be lost in the mists of age and medication, but your presence will be cherished. It may be heart-breaking and soul-burdening to remain a faithful visitor of the old and infirm, but bringing love and change to someone whose only failure has been their arrival at the natural end of their stay on earth will affirm the power of family love, faith and continuity in the noblest way, demonstration.

Alzheimer's Disease

There is a growing awareness of Alzheimer's disease and the devastation it brings to the elderly and the families of its victims. Because of media coverage the alarming numbers of people suffering, and the prolonged agony of many as they watch the steady deterioration of older loved one's mind, spirit and body, the medical-scientific community has launched a concerted effort to find the cause, to understand and to treat this disease.

ADRDA (Alzheimer's Disease and Related Disorders)—see page 187 in the Resources section for address and phone number—is a national organization working on behalf of Alzheimer's victims and their families to create comprehensive programs of research, education, advocacy and patient care assistance through funding and dedicated volunteers. If your loved one is suffering from Alzheimer's, contact this worthy organization for information and support.

Medicare, Medicaid

Keep a photocopy or carbon copy for your records of *each* claim for Medicare payment. Note the date you sent it in and each service received, the date and charge for each service received, and the name of the doctor, clinic or supplier billing you.

When a person covered by Medicare dies, payments will be made directly by Medicare to the hospital, skilled nursing facility, or home health agency where that person died. Ask for a copy of this statement for your records. You will need it at tax time.

If the doctor or medical supply bills are *not accepted* (some doctors and facilities will not work with Medicare), payment is made to the person paying and submitting the bills with proof of payment. These forms should be requested from your local Social Security office, and should include:

1. *Medicare Payment* Form SSA-1490.
2. A Statement Regarding Medicare Payment.
3. A List of Medical Services to Deceased Patient.

Remember, all social services are in the process of revision. You are responsible for keeping current on these changes through your local agency.

Resource-Reference Material for the Elderly

NRTA/AARP
(National Retired Teachers Association for Retired People)
1909 "K" Street
Washington, D.C. 20049

Gerontological Society
One Dupont Circle, #520
Washington, D.C. 20036

National Council of Senior Citizens
1511 "K" Street
Washington, D.C. 20005

Gray Panthers
3708 Chestnut Street
Philadelphia, PA 19104

National Indian Council on Aging, Inc.
PO Box 2088
Albuquerque, NM 87103

National Association for Spanish-Speaking Elderly
(Associacion Nacionale por Personas Mayores)
3875 Wilshire Blvd. #401
Los Angeles, CA 90005

National Center of Black Aged
1730 "M" Street, NW
Washington, D.C. 20036

American Geriatrics Society
10 Columbus Circle
New York, NY 10023

National Council on Aging
1828 "L" Street, NW
Washington, D.C. 20036

American Association of Homes for the Aging
529 14th Street, NW
Washington, D.C. 20004

Urban Elderly Coalition
250 Broadway
New York, NY 10007

National Association of Area Agencies on Aging
c/o Central Bank Building, #350
Huntsville, Alabama 35801

National Senior Citizens Law Center
1709 W. 8th Street
Los Angeles, CA 90017

Legal Services for the Elderly Poor
2095 Broadway
New York, NY 10023

National Continuing Care Directory
AARP Books
Scott, Foresman & Co.
400 S. Edward St.
Mt. Prospect, Ill. 60056
(Distributed by Farrar, Straus & Giroux)

Luckily, medicine, science and social service programs recognize the trauma and drain a child's terminal illness brings to each family member. Doctors, hospitals, clinics, churches, foundations and organizations have formed support groups, information centers and networks to deal with the complications brought on by terminal illness.

Next to finding the best primary care for your child, the most important task is to find the resources *you* need to cope with the problems such an ordeal brings to your family. The best and often the only way to do this is to actively seek out others who are living or have lived the day-to-day grind of caring and coping. The suggestions here come from these people as well as pediatricians, pediatric nurses, and pediatric social workers.

When your child has been diagnosed and you have sought the opinion of other doctors to substantiate the illness, *ask questions.* Ask over and over until you fully understand the illness and what to expect from it. People meeting with you at this time know and understand that your defense mechanisms do not allow you to grasp everything they tell you. Don't be embarrassed to ask them to repeat information or to write it out so that you can absorb it at your own level of understanding. There are clinical aspects of the disease and treatment a layman cannot be expected to understand at first but which, with patience and understanding on the part of the care-givers, can be made clear.

At first during the illness, you will feel isolated, but as time goes on and your understanding becomes clear, you will be included in every facet of the illness *if you express a desire to be a part of the care team.* If you feel excluded, it is your responsibility to make your desires known. Many doctors are in a quandary as to how involved parents want to become with the care of their child. They welcome a frank discussion with parents which includes your assessment of your tolerance and capabilities. If all the parties concerned with providing care and treatment have an open relationship from the outset of an illness, recognizing the limitations and expectations of each toward the other, a viable team can be formed which is helpful to everyone concerned.

CHAPTER · 17

Children

Nothing is more devastating than the terminal illness of a child. When you know a child's life is threatened your emotional upheaval is magnified many times over. The complications within your family can seem insurmountable, and when you realize that death is the final resolution, desperation sets in.

There is a brighter side to this soul-racking dilemma: *hope*. Many formerly terminal childhood diseases have been conquered and controlled in the past decade and many others will be through the constant research of thousands of dedicated doctors and scientists. Hope will be the guiding light for you through the period ahead.

The care and responsibility you face when a child is in a life-threatening illness is manifestly more difficult than can be imagined by those who have not experienced it. It is for this reason that no person or family should ever attempt to "go it alone."

One parent said, "It's like having a bomb go off in the middle of a family. At first you're in such shock, nothing registers. Then reality sets in and you try to pick up the pieces and patch up life as best you can. Everything changes. If you aren't *very* careful, all the relationships within the family and among your friends get warped and jaded. The disease takes over your whole world and—well, if you don't get help for yourself and others in your family, and learn how to cope— how to preserve your sanity and your emotional and physical endurance, more than the child will die . . . the family unit will become terminal."

The support systems that have formed around families suffering through the critical period of a child's illness can help all of you deal with emotional trauma, family stress, fatigue, communication with doctors and other care-givers, financing, pain, medication, and therapies, marital problems, sibling needs and conflicts, school and social needs, psychological problems related to the illness, religious conflicts, societal attitudes, hospital, home, and hospice care, the need for rest and relaxation, ways to deal with home treatment, and all the available information, resource and support systems.

As you can see, the load of care and responsibility is enormous. If, early on in the illness, you force yourself to face and understand that your needs, the needs of the child who is ill, and the needs of other family members *exceed the emotional, physical, and economic resources* of the average family unit, and if you seek help *before crisis*, you will have the reserve necessary to carry on when and if it becomes necessary to call in outside expertise.

And how do you go about finding the necessary resources and support? By assertively seeking it through the many avenues open to all of us. Here is a list of primary resource and information people and places which was suggested by those who work daily with parents of the terminally ill:

1. *Your doctor.* The pediatrician in charge of the patient constantly receives information from local and national organizations dealing with diseases of children and from support groups formed to assist families.
2. *Local and state organizations.* See the Yellow Pages in the telephone directory and the Support, Information and Referral Sources section of this book in Appendix II.
3. *Social workers* in hospitals and the Human Resources office (city, state or federal H.E.W.).
4. *State university hospitals, medical schools, medical centers, specialized clinics, Visiting Nurses Association, health science centers, etc.*

163

5. *Libraries.* Ask to see directories of support groups and organizations.
6. *Churches and synagogues.* Religious organizations have family counseling and support groups. Chaplain's office in the hospital.

If you feel unable to do your own research, ask a friend or family member to help. The support group Candlelighters was formed within the Childhood Cancer Foundation and offers a prime example of the family-oriented organizations making an enormous impact in helping families of cancer patients. Other such groups exist nationwide that are ready and able to help if you ask; it is only a question of being assertive in your search.

Scientific progress may force you to choose between the length of time your child can live and the quality of life to be led. It is a heart-rending dilemma children's doctors constantly face and one you should be prepared to consider. As parents it is your job to recognize that a doctor's training and dedication demand the use of every weapon at his or her disposal to fight death. Sometimes doctors, feeling "damned if they do and damned if they don't," sustain life regardless of the consequences. Recognizing this problem early and preparing for it by deeply considering your own needs and beliefs will help you cope with this crucial issue.

Your decision involves every humanitarian, ethical, religious and moral principle at your disposal. Each element should be weighed and measured against the consideration of what is best for the child and what the ramifications of this decision mean for the parents and the doctors involved. Life can be sustained almost indefinitely. But what would the quality of that life be for the child? It is important that you agree as a family and let the doctor in charge know how you feel.

According to the people who spend their professional lives caring for sick children, these are your responsibilities and duties as parents:

1. Be honest about your emotions, capabilities and limitations. You must learn to enunciate your

164

feelings and acknowledge your need for support and understanding.

2. You must learn to communicate concerns to doctors, nurses, and care-givers.

3. Get training and understanding from people who can show you how to deal with the physical as well as the emotional needs of your child.

4. Deal with honesty in relationships with the patient and other family members. Let them know you are hurting too, share it—but don't wallow in it.

5. Make it *your* job to seek help. The medical and psychological community is ready and willing to assist, but it is expected that those with needs will seek help.

6. Children are more comfortable when their parents are present during treatment. Learn how to steel yourself for discomfort, pain, or fear— remembering that your acceptance and encouragement are vital to the attitude of your child.

7. *You* are your child's advocate. *You* are the key person in every facet of treatment and care. Strong, loving, knowledgeable parents who have made themselves "experts" in active teamwork with professional care-givers are finding an outlet for their love and concern. There will be less frustration when participation and sharing are the modes of operation.

8. As parents you have the right to challenge treatment. You have the right to second and even third and fourth opinions. You have the right to question the validity of prolonging life in a hopeless situation. You have the right to question and the right to expect clear, intelligible answers.

9. Parents *know* intuitively what is best for their child. Insist that this intuition is respected.

10. Expect guilt. It is normal to wonder if perhaps you or your actions contributed to the cause of

the illness of a loved one. Discuss any guilt feelings you have with a person who understands and can help relieve you of this burden.

11. Use all the tools at your disposal: support systems, information, discipline, religion and/or philosophy.

12. Make life good and happy within the limitations placed on you and your family. Seek comfort, normality, relaxation, rest for yourself and your entire family.

13. Each day brings new discoveries and new hope. You can be as brave as you decide to be. It takes practice to be courageous. Allow yourself to fail occasionally, but keep trying.

14. Take your comforts and rest whenever and wherever they are available, but don't allow yourself to be wooed by drugs or alcohol. A healthy body is your best weapon during troubled times. Take care of yourself.

15. Make the time you have with your child *quality* time. Make happy memories; they will be bittersweet but lasting. Make friends along the way. They will buoy you up and share your load. Make time for thinking, praying and resting. This is the hardest battle life will ever bring you. You need all the reserves you can find, but help is there for those who seek it.

Afterword

Bob died at ten minutes before six on the morning of December 5th. He was at home alone with me just as he wished. We had agreed that if the process of dying became too painful (the "process" was a greater fear than death), I would help him end his struggle. I would have helped, but I'm profoundly grateful I was spared that final agony.

Like everyone whose loved one dies, my loss was the greatest, my sorrow the deepest, my spirit the most crumpled. You will feel as I did, I am sure. Your pain will be the axis on which the world turns—for a while.

And then after months of emotional confusion—grief feels like fear, and drunkenness, anesthesia, and isolation—there came a spark, a flash of color in what had been the interminably gray landscape of my world. Hope and feeling and life began to grow. It happens that way to all of us. We begin to realize that although life and living will never be the same, we can accept the change and become accustomed to the vacuum left by the death of the one we loved. Someday we will feel rested, whole, and able to laugh and love again, never quite the way we were before, but enough to know we've met the challenge and have grown in spirit.

All this will happen through natural healing over a period of time but the pain will be less if you understand the process of healing and have knowledge of the important steps of grieving. Don't be too proud or self-centered to seek and accept help. Support groups and books on grief are the sum totals of thousands who have walked through the valley of the shadows. Use them and be grateful.

Remember, each of us who loses a loved one suffers an amputation. We must heal and adapt at our own pace and capacity. Healing will not come by our madly rushing around seeking miracle cures in escape, change, or drugs. Healing comes through introspection, acceptance, and faith.

Take your time. Grieve naturally. Heal naturally. Join the others who have learned to look out from the center of pain and give thanks for the time they had to share life with the one they loved.

Someone once said a writer writes not so much to be understood as to understand. So it has been with me. By sharing others' grief and hurt, by listening to their experiences and realizing that one must accept that which cannot be changed, and by passing important information on to you, I have found we choose either to grow or wither by our response to the loss of a person we love.

It takes time. It takes faith. It takes patience. But in return we receive strength and courage and a sense of at-oneness, a connection with, and an awareness of every human being we meet.

Someday you will sigh and ask as I did:

> "Will I ever see a rainbow
> and not think of him,
> Or feel a wind rift from the river,
> Or watch a moonrise,
> Or sunset?
> Will I ever see a leaf turn silver in the light
> And not think of him?
> Or hear the geese gossip as they settle,
> Or jazz played well,
> Or laughter?
> I think not."

The painful times you've gone through recently will become less sharp as times goes on. You will be able to accept the honest assessment of our existence so simply written thousands of years ago: "For every thing there is a season and a time for every matter under heaven."

Birth, life and death. It is the ultimate trinity all must bear.

Appendix I

Sample Form for
Assignment of Title for Personal Property

Selling Price $_____

For value received, the undersigned hereby sell(s), assign(s), or transfer(s) UNTO [name of purchaser]_____, _____, ADDRESS [number, street, section, apt. no.] _____

the motor vehicle or trailer described on the reverse side of this certificate, and the undersigned hereby warrant(s) the title to said _____ [fill in motor vehicle—boat, etc.] and certifies that at the time of delivery the same is subject to the following liens or encumbrances and none other:

AMOUNT   KIND   DATE   FAVOR OF

Signature of assigner (seller) _____

On this ___ day of _____ , 19__, before me, the subscriber, a Notary Public of _____, personally appeared _____, who made oath in due form of law that the above statements are true.

Witness my hand and notarial seal.

_____
Notary Public for the State of
_____.
My commission expires:_____

Sample Form for Living Will

TO MY FAMILY, MY PHYSICIAN, MY LAWYER AND ALL OTHERS WHOM IT MAY CONCERN:

Death is as much a reality as birth, growth, maturity and old age—it is the one certainty of life. If the time comes when I can no longer take part in decisions for my own future, let this statement stand as an expression of my wishes and directions, while I am still of sound mind.

If at such a time the situation should arise in which there is no reasonable expectation of my recovery from extreme physical or mental disability, I direct that I be allowed to die and not be kept alive by medications, artificial means or "heroic measures." I do, however, ask that medication be mercifully administered to me to alleviate suffering even though this may shorten my remaining life.

This statement is made after careful consideration and is in accordance with my strong convictions and beliefs. I want the directions here expressed carried out to the extent permitted by law. Insofar as they are not legally enforceable, I hope that those to whom this Will is addressed will regard themselves as morally bound by these provisions.

Signed _____ Date_____

Witness _____ Witness _____

Copies of this Will given to: _____

_____

_____

This is a *general* Living Will. If your state honors the Living Will, it may have forms slightly different from this. The *Society for the Right to Die*, 250 West 57th Street, New York, NY 10019, can guide, direct and assist you in finding the proper form of Living Will for the state in which you live. See also Hemlock Society—P.O. Box 66218, Los Angeles, CA 90066, which supports the option of passive or active voluntary euthanasia for the terminally ill.

Letter of Intent

This is a letter which is *not* a Will, but eliminates uncertainty and confusion as to the wishes of the deceased. *This letter does not substitute for a Will and should not be placed in a safety deposit box.* It should be given to the executor of the estate, the next of kin, or a close, trusted friend.

The letter should include:

1. The location of the Will
2. Funeral or burial instructions
3. Location of all important documents
4. Location of safety deposit box and where the keys can be found
5. A list and location of insurance policies (name, number, amount and beneficiary), health, accident and burial policies
6. Pension or stock sharing plans
7. Bank accounts (checking and savings)
8. Stocks and bonds and where they are located
9. Real estate holdings
10. Major properties (personal and business)
11. Instruction and direction on business management
12. Names, addresses and telephone numbers of advisors such as lawyers, insurance agents, clergy, accountants, bankers, etc.
13. Names of close relatives and friends with addresses and telephone numbers
14. A list of how certain personal effects should be dispersed, to whom and by whom
15. Any other requests not included in a Will

Once all the Very Important Papers have been gathered together as suggested on page 105, a Letter of Intent becomes relatively simple. It is a sort of gathering up of loose ends and a chance to express personal desires and preferences that otherwise might go unheeded. It can be a very informal letter, or it can be structured by an attorney. In many cases, it is a simple, dictated statement asking that certain people receive certain personal possessions or that the final disposition of one's body after death be taken care of in a specified manner. It is the sort of thing that solves the problems of who will receive father's watch or mother's wedding ring, which is often the cause of family problems after a Will has been read.

Sample of
Limited Power of Attorney Form

_____ provides _____ limited power of attorney on this _____ day of _____, 19__ .
Knowing my wishes and desires regarding my health care and treatment and the disposition of my real and personal property and remains, _____ shall have the right to act on my behalf and make decisions in these areas should I become physically or mentally incapable of doing so.

This limited power of attorney will be valid until it is revoked by me. I retain the power to revoke it at any time.

I fully understand the contents of this document and fully trust _____ to act in my best interests.

In accepting this power of attorney,_____ agrees to act in good faith and in the best interests of _____.

_____

I accept this power of attorney.

_____

Subscribed and sworn to before me this ____ day of _____, 19__ .

_____
NOTARY PUBLIC

Signed in the presence of the following witnesses:

_____
WITNESS (SIGNATURE)   (PRINT NAME)

ADDRESS OF ABOVE WITNESS
_____

WITNESS (SIGNATURE)   (PRINT NAME)
_____

ADDRESS OF ABOVE WITNESS
_____

Sample of General Form for
Last Will and Testament of

I, _____, of the city of
_____, and state of _____,
being of sound mind, memory, and understanding, declare
this to be my last will and testament, as follows:

1. *Debts and Funeral Expenses.* I direct that all debts
enforceable against my estate, and funeral expenses, be paid
as soon as possible.

2. *Executor and Trustee.* I nominate and appoint_____
_____ as executor and trustee of my estate. My
executor and trustee shall have the full power at his discretion
to do all the things necessary for the liquidation of my estate.

3. *Spouse.* I give and bequeath to my_____
[husband or wife] all my interest in real estate and 50% of all
money that I have in banks, savings and loans, certificates of
deposit, and similar institutions.

4. *Children.* I give and bequeath the following items to
my children. To my son, _____, I give_____
_____.
To my daughter, _____, I give_____
_____. To my
_____, _____, I give_____
_____.

5. *Charity.* I give and bequeath the following items to
charitable organizations. To _____, I give
_____. To_____
_____ I give _____.

6. *Remainder of Estate.* I direct that the remainder of my
estate be sold and that the proceeds be divided as follows:
_____
_____.

173

PAGE ONE APPROVAL:

_____

7. *Death of Beneficiaries.* In the event that any of the beneficiaries named in this will die before me, or at approximately the same time as me, I direct that their children shall take their share, equally. In the event that any of the beneficiaries die before me without leaving children, I direct that the remaining named beneficiaries shall take their share, equally.

8. *Revocation of Other Wills.* I hereby revoke all prior wills, codicils, and testamentary dispositions made by me.

IN WITNESS TO THIS WILL I HAVE SET MY HAND TO THIS WILL THIS ____ DAY OF _____, 19__.

_____

This will, consisting of _____ pages, each bearing the signature of _____, was signed on this date, and declared by _____ to be his last will and testament.

The will was signed in the presence of the following three witnesses:

_____	_____
WITNESS	WITNESS
_____	_____
SIGNATURE	SIGNATURE
_____	_____
ADDRESS	ADDRESS

_____

WITNESS

_____

SIGNATURE

_____

ADDRESS

Sample of
Unlimited Power of Attorney Form

_____ provides _____ full power of attorney on this ____ day of _____, 19__.

_____ shall have the power and the right to sell or assign my real and personal property, to enter into contracts in my name, to withdraw funds from bank and savings accounts in my name, to use my property as he chooses, to enter my safe deposit boxes as he chooses and to do any and all acts as I could do personally.

This power of attorney shall be valid until revoked by me. I shall retain the power to revoke it at any time.

I fully understand the contents of this document and fully trust _____ to act in my best interests.

In accepting this power of attorney,_____ agrees to act in good faith and in the best interests of _____.

_____

I accept this power of attorney.

_____

Subscribed and sworn to before me this _____ day of _____, 19__.

_____
                        NOTARY PUBLIC
Signed in the presence of the following witnesses:

_____
WITNESS (SIGNATURE)   (PRINT NAME)

_____
ADDRESS OF ABOVE WITNESS

_____
WITNESS (SIGNATURE)   (PRINT NAME)

_____
ADDRESS OF ABOVE WITNESS

NOTE: An Unlimited Power of Attorney is a powerful document. Before signing or accepting its responsibilities, be *absolutely sure* you understand all the ramifications, which can be explained only by an attorney familiar with the state laws under which it is written and accepted.

Agreement to Live Together—Sample

1. *Parties.* This agreement is made this ＿＿＿＿＿ day of ＿＿＿＿＿, 19＿, by ＿＿＿＿＿＿＿＿＿＿＿＿＿ and ＿＿＿＿＿＿＿＿＿＿＿＿＿＿ who presently reside in the state of ＿＿＿＿＿＿＿＿＿＿＿.

2. *Relationship.* We wish to live together in a relationship similar to matrimony but do not wish to be bound by the statutory or case-law provisions relating to marriage.

3. *Duration of Relationship.* It is agreed that we will live together for an indefinite period of time subject to the following terms:

4. *Partnership.* We agree that we are a partnership for all purposes;

5. *Common Property.* Any real or personal property acquired during the relationship shall be considered to be owned equally;

PAGE ONE APPROVAL:

＿＿＿＿＿＿＿＿＿＿＿＿＿＿＿＿＿＿

Man

＿＿＿＿＿＿＿＿＿＿＿＿＿＿＿＿＿＿

Woman

6. *Income.* All income of either of us and all our accumulations during the existence of our relationship shall be one fund. Our debts and expenses arising during the existence of our union shall be paid out of this fund. Each of us shall have an equal interest in this sum, an equal right to its management and control, and an equal entitlement to the excess remaining after payment of all debts and expenses;

7. *Abortion.* If the man desires the abortion of any embryo created by us but the woman wants to bear the child, the woman releases the man from any and all legal obligations

of any nature that he might otherwise have by reason of the birth of such a child; and the man must express his disapproval of the birth in writing, signed and notarized and given to the woman at least five months before the birth. The woman shall have the exclusive right to determine whether or not she may have an abortion.

PAGE TWO APPROVAL:

_____

Man

_____

Woman

8. *Children.* Any children born of us shall have the surname _____. If both of us want to have, and do have, a child by our union, the child shall be maintained and supported from our common fund for as long as we live together. We are equally obligated for the support of the child upon termination of our relationship. We shall, upon termination, be equally obligated to spend not less than one-fifth of our respective incomes for the maintenance and education of the child until he/she reaches the age of eighteen.

9. *Child Custody.* Both of us shall have joint custody of any children. The_____ shall have their care
(mother or father)
and control unless otherwise agreed.

10. *Separate Property.* All property listed on the pages attached is made a part of this agreement by this reference. The property belongs to the one under whose name it is listed prior to the making of this agreement. All listed property is and shall continue to be the separate property of the person who now owns it. All property received by either of us by gift or inheritance during our relationship shall be the separate property of the one who receives it.

177

PAGE THREE APPROVAL:

_____
Man

_____
Woman

11. *Termination.* Our relationship may be terminated at the sole will and decision of either of us, expressed by a written notice given to the other.

12. *Modification of this Agreement.* This agreement may be modified by any agreement in writing signed by both parties, with one exception: no modifications may decrease the obligations that we have agreed to undertake regarding any children born of our union.

13. *Breach of Contract.* If either party fails to perform any obligations required by this agreement, that one shall be responsible for all legal expenses incurred by the other in obtaining the performance of those obligations, including those incurred in seeking damages for the breach of this agreement.

14. *Application of Law.* The validity of this agreement shall be determined solely under the laws of the state of _____ as they may from time to time be changed.

SIGNED:

_____
Man

_____
Woman

Instructions
UNIFORM ANATOMICAL GIFT ACT
Donor Form

When properly completed, this form and a similar uniform donor card which will be sent to you when the form is returned, are legal documents in all 50 states.

Return the white copy of this form to The Living Bank as soon as it is completed. Keep the yellow one for your files.

Be sure to have your signature on the form witnessed by two persons of legal age, preferably some of your next of kin so they will be aware of your decision to be an organ donor. At least one parent or legal guardian must sign as a witness if the donor is a minor.

This form is not legal unless two witnesses sign it with the donor in the presence of each other.

You may check either (A) or (B) alone or you may check (C) alone or in addition to either (A) or (B). When you check (C), you are signifying that you wish to donate your body for anatomical study. Acceptance of the body donation depends upon the needs of medical schools at the time of death and cannot be guaranteed.

Willed body programs are full in a number of areas and only pre-registered donors are accepted. If you check (C), it is recommended that you register with a medical school in your area if you wish to donate your body.

Body donations are usually refused if an autopsy has been performed and in cases of contagion or for other medical reasons. If a body donation is refused by the medical school, the family of the deceased is responsible for disposition of the body.

There is no payment made for body or organ and tissue donations. Also, there are no costs to the donor's family for organ donations.

In some cases, body donations can be made in areas away from the place of death if the family will pay transportation costs, which vary.

Organs and/or tissue for transplant must be medically acceptable at the time of death. There are no delays in funeral arrangements. An open casket funeral service can be held if desired.

THE LIVING BANK
P.O. Box 6725
Houston, Texas 77265
In Texas: (713) 528-2971   U.S.A.: 1-800-528-2971

RETURN WHITE COPY TO THE LIVING BANK. KEEP YELLOW COPY FOR YOUR FILES. Your donor card will be sent to you when we receive the white copy of this donor registration form.

To Remember Me

The day will come when my body will lie upon a white sheet neatly tucked under four corners of a mattress located in a hospital busily occupied with the living and the dying. At a certain moment a doctor will determine that my brain has ceased to function and that, for all intents and purposes, my life has stopped.

When that happens, do not attempt to instill artificial life into my body by the use of a machine. And don't call this my deathbed. Let it be called the Bed of Life, and let my body be taken from it to help others lead fuller lives.

Give my sight to the man who has never seen a sunrise, a baby's face or love in the eyes of a woman.

Give my heart to a person whose own heart has caused nothing but endless days of pain.

Give my blood to the teen-ager who was pulled from the wreckage of his car, so that he might live to see his grandchildren play.

Give my kidneys to one who depends on a machine to exist from week to week.

Take my bones, every muscle, every fiber and nerve in my body and find a way to make a crippled child walk.

Explore every corner of my brain. Take my cells, if necessary, and let them grow so that, someday, a speechless boy will shout at the crack of a bat and a deaf girl will hear the sound of rain against her window.

Burn what is left of me and scatter the ashes to the winds to help the flowers grow.

If you must bury something, let it be my faults, my weaknesses and all prejudice against my fellow man.

If, by chance, you wish to remember me, do it with a kind deed or word to someone who needs you.
If you do all I have asked, I will live forever.

Reprinted courtesy of
The Living Bank
P. O. Box 6725
Houston, Texas 77005
(713) 528-2971

Written by Robert N. Test
printed in the Cincinnati Post
reprinted in Reader's Digest
appeared in "Dear Abby's" syndicated
column Decembei

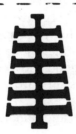

The
Living Bank

P. O. Box 6725 ● Houston, Texas 77265

713/528-2971

(Wats) 1-800-528-2971

Uniform Donor Card

EMERGENCY

Appendix II: Support, Information and Referral Sources

These are names and addresses of associations, organizations, networks and foundations you can contact for information and support during the illness of a loved one. Hospitals, doctors, clergy, and social workers are also good sources for materials and assistance. These associations, organizations and foundations also welcome memorial gifts and donations.

Do It Now Foundation
   Institute for Chemical Survivor
   PO Box 5115
   Phoenix, AZ 85010
   Publications list and catalog of substance abuse information.
The American Lupus Society (Lupus Erythematosus)
   23751 Madison Street
   Torrence, CA 90505
   Funding for research, patient care, and support.
National Lupus Erythematosus Foundation
   5430 Van Nuys Blvd, #206
   Van Nuys, CA 91401

USC-LA County Medical Center and City of Hope publishes leaflets to answer questions. Offers telephone counseling services.

Alliance for Cannabis Therapeutics
Box 23691
Washington, DC 20024
(202) 544-2884
Working to "construct a medically meaningful, ethically correct and compassionate system of regulation which permits the seriously ill to legally obtain cannabis for relief."

Center of Attitudinal Healing
(Children and adult mental health)
19 Main Street
Tiburon, CA 94920
(415) 435-5022
Programs offering attitudinal healing to children and adults suffering life-threatening or catastrophic illness and offering guidance to their families.

American Institute for Research and Education in Naturopathy
7 Porpoise Drive
Centerreach, NY 11720
Supports the rights of those whose legal right to nature-cure health care is denied. Conducts research and training therapy through horticulture. Established college in 1979.

International Naturopathic Association
3519 Thom Blvd
Las Vegas, NV 99106
(213) 479-1945
Research, legal aid, legislation. Directory of professional and naturopathic physicians and hospitals.

American Parkinson Disease Association
116 John Street, #417
New York City, NY 10038
(217) 732-9550
"To alleviate pain and suffering of the Parkinsonian by subsidizing information and referral centers and providing funds for research to find a cure for the disease." Provides counseling for patients and families.

183

Amyotrophic Lateral Sclerosis
  15300 N. Ventura Blvd, #315
  Sherman Oaks, CA 91403
  (213) 990-2151
  Offers help and information to ALS patients and families. Provides ALS-related research at major medical institutions. Referral service.

Arthrogryposis Association
  106 Herkimer Street
  North Bellmore, NY 11710
  (516) 221-6968
  To share information and self-help for victims and care-takers.

Committee to Combat Huntington's Disease
  250 W 57th Street, #2016
  New York City, NY 10017
  (212) 757-0443
  Public and professional education, promotes and supports basic and clinical research, maintains patient service, assists in dealing with social, economic, and emotional problems. Information and referral.

Dysautonomia Foundation
  370 Lexington Avenue, #1504
  New York City, NY 10017
  (212) 889-0300
  Research and referral.

Dystonia Foundation
  425 Broad Hollow Road
  Melville, NY 11746
  (516) 249-7799
  Referral and support for patients with Torsion dystonia and their families.

Friedreich's Ataxia Group in America
  PO Box 11116
  Oakland, CA 94611
  Clearinghouse for information concerning the physical and emotional wellbeing of patients.

Georgia Warm Springs Foundation
  600 Third Avenue, #2500

New York City, NY 10016
(212) 490-3361
Dedicated to treatment and rehabilitation of stroke, arthritis and other conditions.

Muscular Dystrophy Association
810 Seventh Avenue
New York City, NY 10019
(212) 586-0808
Local, national and international service for diagnosis, medical evaluation, orthopedic appliances, physical therapy, flu shots, recreation for victims and families.

Myasthenia Gravis Foundation
15 E 26th Street
New York City, NY 10010
(212) 889-8157
Supports low-cost diagnostic and treatment clinics, low-cost medication bank and public information services.

National ALS Foundation (Lou Gehrig's disease)
185 Madison Avenue
New York City, NY 10016
(212) 679-4016
Supports ALS clinics at Mount Sinai Center, NY; University of Chicago Medical Center, Chicago, IL. Provides equipment for patients when available, makes necessary contacts for patients, arranges autopsies for research. Offers family counseling and publishes information.

National Committee for Research in Neurological and Communicative Disorders
1120 20th Street, #S-520
Washington, DC 20036
Public and governmental information re: neurological and communicative disorders and strokes.

National Huntington's Disease Association
1182 Broadway
New York City, NY 10019
(212) 684-2781
Provides guidance and assistance to patients and their families in areas of emotional, social, medical and physical needs. Publishes information.

National Association of Children's Hospitals and Related Institutes
1601 Concord Pike, #34
Wilmington, DE 19803
(302) 571-0882
Publishes guide to children's hospitals annually.

National Association of Patients on Hemodialysis
505 Northern Blvd
Great Neck, NY 11021
(516) 482-2720
Association to educate patients and public, publish supportive material and promote donor programs.

National Kidney Foundation
Two Park Avenue
New York City, NY 10016
(212) 889-2210

Council of Teaching Hospitals
One Dupont Circle, NW, #200
Washington, DC 20036
(202) 828-0490
Directory of Education Service Programs—associated with American Medical Colleges.

American Healthcare Association
1200 15th Street
Washington, DC 20005
See State Health Care Associations in Yellow Pages.

National Hemophilia Foundation
19 West 34th Street, #1204
New York City, NY 10001
(213) 563-0211

Leukemia Society of America
800 Second Avenue
New York City, NY 10017
Also: 211 E. 43rd Street
New York City, NY 10017
Information and assistance for needy patients.

National Leukemia Association
Roosevelt Field—Lower Concourse
Garden City, NY 14550

Garden City, NY 14550
Research and awareness, provides financial aid to patients and families.

National Rare Blood Club
c/o Association Health Foundation
164 Fifth Avenue
New York City, NY 10010
(212) 243-8037
Volunteers 18–65 years of age with rare blood who are physically able to donate blood for those in need. Publishes a directory.

Action Against Burns
c/o Joan Hand
PO Box 239
Charlestown, MA 02129
Mutual aid for burn victims and families.

American Burn Association
New York Hospital–Cornell Medical Center
525 E 68th Street, Room F 0758
New York City, NY 10021
Information on improved care and treatment of burn patients.

Hemlock Society
PO Box 66218
Los Angeles, CA 90066
(213) 391-1971
A group supporting the right of a terminally ill patient to terminate his/her own life.

Society for the Right to Die
250 West 57th Street
New York City, NY 10017
Information, forms in support of dying with dignity.

Alzheimer's Disease and Related Disorders Association
292 Madison Avenue, 8th Floor
New York City, NY 10017
(212) 683-2868
Alzheimer's disease and multi-infarct dementia research, aid in diagnosis, improved treatment, identification of cause, and support system.

Hotline: 1-800-621-0379
Support and information.

Saint Jude Children's Research Hospital
539 Lane Avenue
Memphis, TN 38105
(901) 522-9733
Treats children of all races and creeds without charge and conducts research on catastrophic children's diseases.

Bay Area Cryonics Society
7710 Huntridge Lane
Cupertino, CA 95014
Interested in the practice of freezing diseased bodies and bringing the bodies back to life when a cure for the disease has been discovered.

American Diabetes Association
One West 48th Street
New York City, NY 10020
Information, referrals, support.

American Diabetes Association
Two Park Avenue
New York City, NY 10016
(See local and state listings.)

Independent Citizens Research Foundation for the Study of Degenerative Diseases
PO Box 97
Ardsley, NY 10502
Publishes information of aids and assistance to those who are closely affected by a degenerative disease.

Airlifeline (emergency aid)
1005 Eighth Street, #302
Sacramento, CA 95814
(916) 442-6230
Voluntary association of pilots, physicians, corporations and interested individuals established to provide a network of air transportation for human organs, medical supplies, personnel, and blood in medical emergencies.

American Foundation for Alternative Health Care
25 Landfield Avenue
Monticello, NY 12701

188

(914) 794-8181

Referral service for alternative healthcare practitioners.

Center for Medical Consumers Health and Care Information

237 Thompson Street

New York City, NY 10012

To encourage people to make a critical evaluation of all information received from health professionals and to use medical services more selectively and to understand the limitations of modern medicine.

Biofeedback Society of America

UCMC, #268

4200 E. 9th Avenue

Denver, CO 80262

Will help locate specialists in biofeedback for pain control.

Cobley's Anemia Foundation

Graybar Bldg, #1644

420 Lexington Avenue

New York City, NY 10017

(212) 687-1564

Selects donations of blood and money; distributes blood and therapy materials at a reduced charge to victims of disease.

Sunshine Foundation (children)

2842 Normandy Drive

Philadelphia, PA 19154

(215) 743-2660

Fulfills wishes of chronic or terminally ill children.

Variety Clubs International (children)

58 W 58th Street, #23-C

New York City, NY 10019

(212) 751-8600

Sponsors charity programs for children, including hospitalization, special treatment centers, etc.

Children's Blood Foundation

342 Madison Avenue

New York City, NY 10017

(212) 687-1564

Operates in NY Hospital—Cornell Medical Center. Provides diagnosis and treatment for children suffering leukemia, hemophilia, hemorrhagia of newborn, thalassemia, sickle cell and other anemias.

National Spinal Cord Injury Foundation
369 Elliot Street
Newton Upper Falls, MA 02164
Supports research, encourages treatment system, assists individuals and peer consultation. Library and referral system.

Assn of Medical School Pediatric Department Chairmen
c/o Jean A. Cortner, M.D.
Children's Hospital of Philadelphia
Philadelphia, PA 19104
(215) 387-6095
Made up of chairmen of the departments of pediatrics of each accredited medical school in the U.S. and Canada, and cooperates with other pediatric groups nationally (therefore should have a directory of pediatric medical help).

City of Hope
208 W 8th Street
Los Angeles, CA 90014
Treatment, research, medical education in catastrophic diseases. Free patient care based on physician's referral.

American Lung Association
1740 Broadway
New York City, NY 10019
(212) 245-8000
Local, state and national groups. Information and referral.

National Jewish Hospital/National Asthma Center
3800 E. Colfax Avenue
Denver, CO 80206
(303) 388-4461
Accepts patients of all ages through physician's referral. Specializes in difficult diagnosis and treatment. Disseminates information.

National Rey's Syndrome Foundation
509 Rosemont
Byran, OH 43506
(419) 636-2679
Provides funds for research and care. Supports and guides families. Publishes information.

190

National Rey's Syndrome Foundation
8293 Homestead Road
Benzonia, MI 49616
(616) 882-5521
Provides support and information to Rey's Syndrome patients and families.

National Multiple Sclerosis Society
205 E. 42nd Street
New York City, NY 10021
(212) 986-3240
Research, services and aids for patients with MS and their families.

National Parkinson Foundation
1501 NW 9th Avenue
Miami, FL 33136
(305) 324-0156
Supports National Parkinson Institute, which provides diagnosis, treatment, care, rehabilitation and literature.

Parkinson Disease Foundation
William Black Research Bldg
Columbia Presbyterian Medical Center
640 168th Street
New York City, NY 10032
(212) 923-4700
Prepares and distributes information on patient care and rehabilitation, including a list of where treatment is available. Supports a brain bank for anatomical research.

United Parkinson Foundation
220 State Street, Room 1710
Chicago, IL 60604
(312) 922-9734
Assembles and publishes reliable information of symptoms, medication and therapy for Parkinson's disease and related illnesses. Assists patient and families through medical referrals and education.

Concerned Relatives of Nursing Home Patients
3137 Fairmount Blvd
Cleveland Heights, OH 44118
(216) 321-0403
Disseminates information on nursing homes to consumers,

191

advises families and social service workers on nursing home placement, Medicaid, Medicare, etc. Accepts grievances.

National Hospice Organization
1311-A Dolly Madison Blvd
McLean, VA 22101
(703) 356-6770

National Hospice Organization
301 Maple Avenue, W
Tower Suite #506
Vienna, VA 22180

United Osomy Association
2001 W. Beverly Blvd
Los Angeles, CA 90057
(213) 413-5510
Support groups exchange of practical information. 600 chapters nationwide.

National Committee on Treatment of Intractable Pain
PO Box 34571
Washington, DC 20034
(301) 983-1710
Endorses British concept of care for terminally ill (hospice) and has a clearing house for information regarding pain control and alternative care for the terminal patient.

Herpetics Engaged in Living Productively (H.E.L.P.)
Box 100
Palo Alto, Ca 94302
Support and information.

American Social Health Association
260 Sherman Avenue, #307
Palo Alto, CA 94306
(415) 321-5134
National voluntary health agency provides resources to local communities. Referrals, support for V.D. patients and problems. Hotline: 1-800-227-8922.

American Medical Association
PO Box 821
New York City, NY
Ask for specific information.

American Red Cross
See local chapter for training and information.

Medical Health Association
  1800 N. Kent Street
  Arlington, VA 22209
  Information, referrals.
Mental Health Materials Center
  410 Park Avenue South
  New York City, NY 10016
  Ask for specific material and local support group.
National Easter Seal Society for Crippled Children and Adults
  2033 W. Ogden Avenue
  Chicago, ILL 60612
  Information.
United Cerebral Palsy Association
  66 East 34th Street
  New York City, NY 10016
  Information and referrals.
Cystic Fibrosis Foundation
  600 Executive Blvd
  Rockville, MD 20852
  (301) 881-9130
  Over 125 care centers nationally, support groups and referrals.
Cystic Fibrosis Center
  3379 Peachtree Road, NE
  Atlanta, GA 30326
  Information and referrals.
National Genetic Foundation
  9 West 57th Street
  New York City, NY 10019
  Information.
Epilepsy Foundation of America
  1828 "L" Street, NW, #406
  Washington, DC 20036
  Information.
American Hospital Association
  840 N. Lake Shore Drive
  Chicago, IL 60611
  Information and directory.
National Tay-Sachs and Allied Diseases Association
  122 East 42nd Street

New York City, NY 10017
Information and referrals.
American Osteopathic Association
212 Ohio Street
Chicago, IL 60611
Shanti Project
c/o Charles Garfield
1314 Addison
Berkeley, CA 94702
Counseling of the terminally ill and recently bereaved. Part
of a national network.

Heart Diseases

American Heart Association
7320 Greenville Avenue
Dallas TX 72531
(214) 750-5300
Councils having resource material on: arteriosclerosis, car-
diopulmonary diseases, cardiovascular surgery, circulation,
clinical cardiology, epidemiology, high blood pressure research, kidney in cardiovascular disease, stroke, thrombosis.
Heart Disease Research Foundation
50 Court Street
Brooklyn, NY 11201
(212) 649-9003
Answers questions from the public and professionals; supplies available educational material on cardiovascular diseases and research.
International Bundle Branch Block Assn (Heart)
6631 W 83rd Street
Los Angeles, CA 90045
(213) 670-9132
Answers inquiries, shares information and research material.

Cancer

American Cancer Society
Public Education

777 Third Avenue
New York City, NY 10017
See also local chapters.

International Foundation for Cancer Research
7315 Wisconsin Avenue, #322-W
Bethesda, MD 20014
Vitamin C therapy and radiofrequency treatment.

One/Fourth, The Alliance for Cancer Patients and Their Families
36 Wabash, #700
Chicago, IL 60603
(312) 346-1414
(One out of four Americans have or will have cancer.) Seeks to address the physical, emotional, social and economic problems created by cancer. Supports the patient's right to know all treatment options available and right to comprehensive pain relief.

United Cancer Council
1803 N Meridan Street
Indianapolis, IN 46202
(317) 923-6490
A federation of independent cancer agencies receiving support from United Way of Giving.

International Assn of Cancer Victims and Friends
7740 W Manchester Avenue, #110
Playa Del Rey, CA 90291
(213) 822-5032
Encourages and supports independent research on cancer therapies, to disseminate information on "non-toxic" chemotherapies, educate on nutrition in relation to cancer and carcinogens in food and the environment. Works directly with patients on a local level and provides a number of total services.

Reach for Recovery
(See American Cancer Society—support group)

Breast Cancer Advisory Center
PO Box 224
Kensington, MD 20795
Referral information.

195

The Breast Cancer Digest (1978)
National Cancer Institute
Office of Cancer Communications
Bethesda, MD
(DHEW Publications #NIH79-1691)
Committee for Freedom of Choice in Cancer Therapy
146 Main Street, #408
Los Altos, CA 94022
(415) 948-9475
Supports freedom of choice for cancer therapy which shows evidence of efficacy and to prohibit interference of government or any third party in the relationship between an informed patient and his physician. Directs people and questions concerning cancer therapy to physicians in their area.

AIDS

Gay Men's Health Crisis Hotline
Box 274
132 West 24th Street
New York, New York 10011
Gay and Lesbian Advocates and Defenders
600 Washington
Boston, MA 02111
Publisher of: *Lesbian and Gay Attorneys' Referral Directory*
National Gay Task Force
80th Fifth Avenue
New York City, New York 10011
(800) 221-7044
(212) 741-5800
Support, information, referrals.
U.S. Department of Health and Human Services
Public Health Service
Washington, DC 20201
(800) 342-AIDS
(202) 245-6867 (collect calls accepted from Alaska or Hawaii) (202) 646-8182 (if calling from DC)
Information and referrals.

196

Center for Disease Control/AIDS Activity
1600 Clifton Road, NE
Atlanta, GA 30333
(404) 329-3311
AIDS Bibliography
National Institute of Allergy and Infectious Disease
National Institute of Health
9000 Rockville Pike
Bethesda, MD 20205
Updated monthly.
Gay Men's Health Crisis
Frederico Gonzales, Director
Department of Education
PO Box 274
132 West 24th Street
New York City, NY 10011
Hotline: (212) 807-6655
Medical answers about AIDS, information, Q & A.
Make Today Count
See Yellow Pages for your local chapter.
AIDS/KS National Foundation
54 10th Street
San Francisco, CA 94103
(415) 626-8784
Publisher of: *AIDS: A Research and Clinical Bibliography*, 3rd ed.
Canadian Gay Archives
Attn: Alan V. Miller
Box 639, Station A
Toronto, Ontario
Canada M5W 162
Publisher of: *Gays and Acquired Immune Deficiency Syndrome*, 3rd ed.
Gay Medical Association
Two Lord Napier Place
Upper Mall
London W6 9UB
United Kingdom
GMA Information Sheets published monthly

197

AIDS Media Reports
  Hall-Carpenter Archives
  34 South Molton Street
  London WY 2BP
  United Kingdom
National Library of Medicine
  Literature Search Program
  Reference Section
  8600 Rockville Pike
  Bethesda, MD 20209
AIDS Project/LA
  937 North Cole Avenue, Suite #3
  Los Angeles, CA 90038
  (213) 817-1284
  Publisher of: *Acquired Immune Deficiency Syndrome,* Vol. I
  and II

Organ Donor Programs

Contact local or state organ procurement programs through
doctor, hospital, medical school, Lion's Sight Foundation, Inc.
or other sponsoring organizations.
Eye Bank for Sight Restoration
  210 E 64th Street
  Houston, TX 77005
  (212) 838-9155
  Information center and registry created to help persons
  who, upon death, wish to donate part or all of their bodies
  for the purpose of transplantation, therapy, medical
  research or anatomical studies. *Donor Registration Form
  and a Uniform Donor Card are the only legal documents under
  the Uniform Anatomical Gift Act which have been passed in
  every state.* (See also Lions Sight Foundation, Inc.)
The Living Bank
  PO Box 6725
  Houston, TX 77265
  (800) 528-2971
  Will put you in contact with local donor procurement
  programs.

American Society for Artificial Internal Organs
PO Box 777
Boca Raton, FL 33432

Healing

Spiritual Frontiers Fellowship (S.F.F.)
10819 Winner Road
Independence, MO 64052
An organization dedicated to bring spiritual healing back to the churches. Will help you find local chapter and recommend healers.

American Healing Association (Holistic)
Box 6311, Yucca Street
Los Angeles, CA 90028
(213) 841-5663
Advances belief that all people have the ability to grow in spirit, mind and body and that the healer is a facilitator toward this goal. Referral service, resources through which healers may exchange information and techniques.

American Holistic Medical Association
6932 Little River Turnpike
Annandale, VA 22003
(703) 642-5880
Defines seven basic subject areas in holistic medicine: acupuncture, environmental medicine, neuromuscular integration, nutrition, physical exercise, self-regulation and spiritual awareness. Referrals.

Association for Holistic Health
PO Box 9532
San Diego, CA
(714) 275-2694
Publishes directory and newsletter.

Spiritual-Religious Network

Unity
Unity Village, MO
(816) 524-7414

Human Unity Councils
3005 Waterdale Drive
Loveland, CO 80537
(303) 667-1219
Church of Religious Science
3201 West 6th Street
Los Angeles, CA
(213) 388-2181
Spiritual Frontiers Fellowship
10819 Winner Road
Independence, MO 64052
(816) 254-8585
Check Yellow Pages for "Dial-a-Prayer" and classified ads. Ask your clergy for your denominational support group, information center and 24-hour help-line (hot line) telephone number.

Addendum

Family Service Association of America
44 E. 33rd Street
New York City, NY 10010
Family Life Bureau
National Catholic Welfare Conf.
1312 Massachusetts Avenue, NW
Washington, DC 20025
Department of Family Life
National Council of Churches of Christ of U.S.A.
475 Riverside Drive
New York City, NY 10027
National Council of Family Relations
1219 University Avenue, SE
Minneapolis, MN 55414
Continental Association of Funeral or Memorial Societies
50 E. Van Buren Street
Chicago, IL 60605
Gerontological Society
One Dupont Circle
Washington, DC 20036

American Lung Association
  1740 N. Broadway
  New York City, NY 10019
Center for Death Education and Research
  Dept. of Sociology
  University of Minnesota
  Minneapolis, MN 55455
Society of Compassionate Friends

Ars Moriendi
  3601 Locust Walk
  Philadelphia, PA 19083
  Information and membership: graceful death, health and human values.
Equinox Institute
  Melvin J. Krant
  11 Clinton Street
  Brookline, MA 02146
  Information and consultation on the dying and their care; help for their surviving loved ones.
Widow to Widow Program
  Laboratory of Community Psychiatry
  58 Fernwood Road
  Boston, MA 02115
  Mutual help—local program.
Administration on Aging
  Dept. of Health, Education and Welfare
  Washington, DC 20201
National Council on Aging
  1828 "L" Street, NW
  Washington, DC 20036
State Office on Aging
  (in the capital city of your state)
National Cancer Programs
  Office of Public Affairs
  Bethesda, MD 20014

Appendix III: Helpful Reading

Alsop, Stewart
  Stay of Execution: A Short Memoir
  J.B. Lippincott
Alvarez, A.
  The Savage God: A Study of Suicide
  Bantam, Random House
Barnard, Christiaan *Good Life Good Death: A Doctor's Case for Euthanasia and Suicide*
  Prentice Hall
Baer, Louis Shattuck, M.D.
  Let the Patient Decide: A Doctor's Advice to Older Persons
  Westminster Press
Battin, Pabst M. and David J. Mayo
  Suicide: The Philosophical Issues
  St. Martin's Press
Battin, Resnick and Lettieri (ed.)
  Prediction of Suicide
  Charles Press, Philadelphia, 1974
Becker, Ernest
  The Denial of Death
  The Free Press, New York, 1973
Bradford, Robert W. with Mike Culbert
  Now That You Have Cancer: General Outline of All Alternative Cancer Treatments
  Choice Publications, 1977

Brown, Tom
  Jeanette: A Memoire
  Lester and Orpen Pub., Toronto
Caine, Lynn
  Widow
  Morrow & Co., Inc., 1974; Bantam, 1975
Cooper, Gary L.
  The Stress Check
  1980 (ISBN 0-13-852640-0)
  (paperback: ISBN 0-13-852632-X)
Colgrove, Melba, Harold Bloomfield and Peter MacWilliams
  How to Survive the Loss of a Love
  Leo Press, 1976
Cousins, Norman
  Anatomy of an Illness as Perceived by the Patient
  W. W. Norton
Covici
  21 Delightful Ways to Commit Suicide
Cutter, F.
  Coming to Terms with Death
  Nelson Hall, Chicago, 1974
Dempsey, David
  The Way We Die: An Investigation of Death and Dying in America
  McGraw-Hill
Dohrendwend, Barbara S. and Bruce D.
  Stressful Life Events
  Wiley, Interscience (LC 74-6369; ISBN 0-471-21753-0)
Downing, A. B. and Peter Owen
  Euthanasia and the Right to Death
  Humanity Press, London
Durkheim, Emile
  Suicide: A Study in Sociology
  (paperback) Free Press
Epstein, Samuel S., M.D.
  The Politics of Cancer
  Sierra Club Press, San Francisco
Feifel, Herman (ed.)
  The Meaning of Death
  McGraw-Hill

Fletcher, Joseph
  Morals and Medicine
  Beacon, Boston
Gerson, Max, M.D.
  A Cancer Therapy: Results of 50 Cases (3rd ed.)
  Totality Books, Delmar, CA, 1977
Gill, Derek
  Quest: The Life of Elizabeth Kubler-Ross
  Harper Row
Glover, Jonathan
  Causing Death and Saving Lives
  Penguin Books
Gordon, Arthur.
  A Touch of Wonder.
  Flemming Revell Company, Old Tappan, N.J., 1974
Gorer, G.
  Death, Grief and Mourning
  Cresset Press, London, 1965
Grof, Stanislau, M.D. and Joan Halifax, Ph.D.
  The Human Encounter with Death
  Dutton
Grollman, Earl A.
  Concerning Death: A Practical Guide for Living
  Beacon Press
Gunderson, E.K.E. and R.H. Rahe
  Life, Stress and Illness
  Chas. C. Thomas, Springfield, 1974
Heifetz, Milton D. with Chas. Mangel
  The Right to Die
  G.P. Putnam and Son: New York (Berkeley Medallion Book, 1975)
Howe, Herbert M.
  Do Not Go Gentle
  W.W. Norton, 1980
Derek, Humphry
  Jean's Way
  Hemlock Society
Janis, Irving L.
  Psychological Stress

Academy Press, 1974 (ISBN 0-12-380750-6)
Stress and Frustration.
Harcourt-Brace. (paperback: ISBN 0-15-583942-X)
Jampolsky, Gerald G.
Love Is Letting Go of Fear
Celestial Arts

_____

Teach Only Love
Bantam, New York, 1983
Kavanaugh, Robert E.
Facing Death
Nash Publishing, Los Angeles, 1972
Kennedy, Betty
Gerhard: A Love Story
Totem Books, Toronto
Klein, Aaron E.
Medical Tests and You
Grosset & Dunlap, New York
Krant, M.J.
Dying and Dignity
Chas. C. Thomas, Springfield, 1974
Kubler-Ross, Elizabeth
Death, the Final Stage of Growth
Prentice-Hall, Englewood Cliffs, 1975

_____

On Children and Dying
The Macmillan Company, New York, 1983

_____

On Death and Dying
The Macmillan Company, New York, 1969
_____and Mel Warshaw
To Live Until We Say Goodbye
Prentice Hall
Kushner, Harold S.
When Bad Things Happen to Good People
Schocken Books, New York, 1981
Kushner, Rose
Why Me?
Signet, New York, 1977

LeShan, Edna
  Learning to Say Goodbye When a Parent Dies
  Avon
LeShan, Lawrence
  You Can Fight for Your Life
  Evans and Co., 1977
Levin, Arthur, M.D.
  Talk Back to Your Doctor
  Doubleday, Garden City, NY, 1975
Linderman, Erich
  Beyond Grief
  Jason Aronson, New York
Liss, Robert E.
  Fading Rainbow
Maguire, Daniel C.
  Death by Choice
  Schocken Books, 1978
Mair, George B., M.D., F.R.C.S., F.R.R.P., F.R.S.G.S.
  How to Die with Dignity
  Scottish Exit, Edinburgh, 1973
Mannes, Marya
  Last Rights
  New American Library, 1973
Marx, Paul Rev.
  Death Without Dignity: Killing for Mercy
  Liturgical Press, 1978
Miller, Jack Silvey
  The Healing Power of Grief
  Crossroad Books, Seabury Press
Mitchell, Paige
  Act of Love
  Bantam
Monat, Alan and Rich S. Lazarus
  Stress and Coping
  (anthology: ISBN 0-685-75644-0: paperback: ISBN 0-685-75645-9)
Moody, Raymond, Jr., M.D.
  Life After Life
  Stackpole

Morgan, Ernest
A Manual of Death Education and Simple Burial
Celo Press
Morris, Sarah
Grief and How to Live with It
Grosset and Dunlap, New York
Moss, Ralph
The Cancer Syndrome
Grove Press, New York, 1980
Osgood, Donald
Pressure Points: How to Deal with Stress
Christian Herald (LC 78-5675; paperback: ISBN
0-915684-59-4).
Owen, Peter
*Euthanasia and the Right to Death: The Case for Voluntary
Euthanasia*
London
Park, Clara Clarborne with Leon N. Shapiro, M.D.
You Are Not Alone
Little, Brown, Boston/Toronto, 1976
Parkes, Colin Murray
Bereavement
International University Press, New York, 1972
Pelletier, Kenneth
Mind as Healer, Mind as Slayer
Dell Publishing Co., New York, 1977
Pincus, Lily
Death and the Family: The Importance of Mourning
Pantheon Books, 1975
Portwood, Doris
Commonsense Suicide: The Final Right
Dodd-Mead
Quinlan, Joseph and Julia with Battelle
Karen Ann: The Quinlans Tell Their Story
Bantam
Rollin, Betty
First You Cry
Signet Books, New York

Last Wish

Roman, Jo
Exit House: Choosing Suicide as an Alternative
Seaview Books
Roman, Mel and Sara Blackburn
Family Secrets: The Experience of Emotional Stress
Times Books (LC 77-87834; ISBN 0-8129-0776-0)
Rossman, Parker
Hospice: Creating New Models of Care for the Terminally Ill
Fawcett-Columbia
Rubin, Theodore I.
The Angry Book
Macmillan, New York
Russell, Ruth O.
Freedom to Die: A Moral and Legal Aspect
Human Science Press
Ryan, Cornelius and Kathryn Morgan Ryan
A Private Battle
Seaview Books
Schiff, Harriet S.
The Bereaved Parent
Crown Publishers, Inc., New York, 1977
Selye, H.
Stress in Health and Disease
(ISBN 0-407-98510-7).

————————.

The Stress of Life
McGraw-Hill (ISBN 0-07-056212-1).
Shneidman, Edwin S.
Death: Current Perspectives
Mayfield, Palo Alto, CA, 1980

————————

Voices of Death: Letters, Diaries, etc.
Harper & Row, New York, 1980
Simonton, O. Carl, M.D., S. Mathew Simonton and Jas. Creighton
Getting Well Again: A Step-by-Step Self-Help Guide to Overcoming Cancer for Patients and Their Families
J.P. Tarcher, Inc.

Smith, Harrison and Robert Hass
To Be or Not to Be
New York, 1933
Stearns, Kaiser Ann
Living Through Personal Crisis
The Thomas More Press, Chicago, 1984
Stoddard, Sandol
The Hospice Movement: A Better Way of Caring for the Dying
Stein and Day
Stuart, Mary E.
To Bend Without Breaking: Stress How to Deal With It
Abingdon (LC 77-6797; paperback: ISBN 0-687-42160-8)
Szasz, Thos
Ceremonial Chemistry
Anchor Press
Thomas, Susan
What to Do, Know and Expect When a Loved One Dies
Wertenbaker, L.
Death of a Man
Random House
West, Jessamyn
The Woman Said Yes
Harcourt Brace
Weisman, Avery D.
On Dying and Denying: A Psychiatric Study of Terminality
Behavioral Publishing
Wohl, Stanley, M.D.
The Medical Industrial Complex
Harmony Books (Crown Pub.) 1984

References and Directories

The Cancer Syndrome
Ralph Moss
Economic factors in cancer treatment, historic background, laetrile, hydrozine sulfate, Dr. Burton's immunological methods, vitamin C, etc.
Cancer: The Wayward Cell: Its Origins, Nature and Treatment

209

Richards, Victor, M.D.
University of California Press, 2nd ed., 1978
Caring: A Family Guide to Managing the Alzheimer's Patient at Home
Cost: $7.00
Payable to: Fund for Aging Services, Inc.,
Alzheimer's Resource Center,
280 Broadway,
New York, NY 10007
Clinical Toxicology of Commercial Products
Gosselin, Hodge, Smith and Gleason
Williams & Wilkins
The Essential Guide to Prescription Drugs
Jas. W. Long, M.D.
Harper & Row, New York, 1980
Profiles drugs, contains generic prescription and over-the-counter drugs, how drugs work, possible side effects.
Justifiable Euthanasia: A Manual for Physicians
P. V. Admirall, M.D.
Netherlands Voluntary Euthanasia Society, Amsterdam, 1981
The Merck Manual of Diagnosis and Therapy
Merck and Co., Rahway, N.J.
The New Handbook of Prescription Drugs
Birack, Richard, M.D. and Fred Fox, M.D.
Ballantine Books, New York
The Pharmacological Basis of Therapeutics
Goodman and Gillman
Macmillan, 1980
Re: toxicology
Physicians' Desk Reference
Published by pharmaceutical industry and given free to physicians—can be found in most libraries.
Strike Back at Cancer: What to Do and Where to Go for the Best Medical Care
Rapaport, Stephan A.
Lists all the qualified cancer specialists in the country, major cancer treatment centers and current medical treatments.

Toxicology: The Basic Science of Poisons
  Cassarett and Doull
  Macmillan, 1980
The Tragedy of Alzheimer's
  Danforth, Art
  Pine Mt. Press, Falls Church VA, 1985
The User Misuse of Sleeping Pills: A Clinical Guide
  W.B. Mendelson, M.D.
  Plenum Medical Book Co., New York/London, 1980
What to Know About the Treatment of Cancer
  Anker, Vincent, M.D.
  Madrona Publishers, Seattle, WA, 1984

Index

Action Against Burns, 187
Administration on Aging, 201
ADRA Alzheimer's Disease,
    187–88
ADRDA (Alzheimer's Disease
    and Related Disorders
    Association), 158, 187
*Advocate's Guide to Hill-Burton
    Uncompensated and
    Community Clearinghouse*,
    101–2
after death, 167–68
Agreement to Live Together
    (sample form), 176–78
AIDS (acquired immune
    deficiency syndrome), 99,
    148–52
    crisis in, 152
    information sources, 151–52,
        196–98
    visiting friend with, 150–51
AIDS Bibliography, 197
AIDS/KS National Foundation,
    197
AIDS Media Reports, 198
AIDS Project/LA, 198
Airlifeline, 188
Alliance for Cannabis
    Therapeutics, 183
Alzheimer's disease, 157–58,
    187–88
Alzheimer's Disease and
    Related Disorders
    Association (ADRDA), 158,
    187

American Association of Homes
    for the Aging, 159
American Bar Association, 116
American Burn Association, 187
American Cancer Society, 56,
    63, 96, 194–95
American College of Nursing
    Home Administrators, 87
American Diabetes Association,
    188
American Foundation for
    Alternative Health Care,
    188–89
American Geriatrics Society,
    159
American Healing Association,
    199
American Healthcare
    Association, 87, 186
American Heart Association,
    194
American Holistic Medical
    Association, 199
American Hospital Association,
    193
American Institute for Research
    and Education in
    Naturopathy, 183
American Lung Association,
    190, 201
American Lupus Society, 182
American Medical Association,
    192
American Osteopathic
    Association, 194

American Parkinson Disease
Association, 183
American Red Cross, 56, 192
American Social Health
Association, 192
American Society for Artificial
Internal Organs, 199
American Way of Death, The
(Mitford), 138
Amyotrophic Lateral Sclerosis,
184, 185
anger, 20–23, 31
hiding of, 21–23
at ill person, 20
reaction to, 32–33
Application for Search of Census
Records, 109
Ars Moriendi, 201
Arthrogryposis Association, 184
Assignment of Title for Personal
Property, 169
Associacion Nacionale por
Personas Mayores, 159
Association for Holistic Health,
199
Association of Medical School
Pediatric Department
Chairmen, 190
Attorney General, state, 102
attorneys:
cost of, 106–7
hiring of, 116
information for, 116–17
selection of, 106–7

bank accounts, 110–11, 121
baptismal certificates, 109
Bay Area Cryonics Society, 188
"Beatitudes for Aging," 153
behavior of patient:
indifferent, 33–34
negative patterns of, 40
observation of, 32
withdrawal, 33
Better Business Bureau, 86, 134
Bible, 52, 109
Biofeedback Society of
America, 189

birth certificates, 109
boredom, 23–24
Breast Cancer Advisory Center,
195
Breast Cancer Digest, 196
brokerage firms, 111
Buddy Training Manual
(GHMC), 152
burns, 187

caffeine, 46–47
California Skilled Nursing
Facilities Regulation,
154–56
Canadian Gay Archives, 197
cancer, 194–96
Candlelighters, 57–58, 164
car care, 60
care-givers:
education by, 28
gifts for, 60–61
hiring of, 95
hiring help for, 62–63
lightening burden of, 59–63
caskets, 132
Catholic churches, 109
cemeteries, 133
lots in, 134–35
service charges, 133
Census Bureau, U.S., 109
Center for Attitudinal Healing,
183
Center for Death Education and
Research, 201
Center for Disease Control/AIDS
Activity, 197
Center for Medical Consumers
Health and Care
Information, 189
cerebral palsy, 193
Certified Public Accountant
Organization, 116
changes, 17, 27–42
decision-making and, 29
information in dealing with,
28–32
in personality, 30–33
physical and environmental, 29

changes (*cont.*)
  in response to situation,
    27–28
  social and interpersonal,
    40–41
checking accounts, 110
child care, 60
  in hospitals, 80
Childhood Cancer Foundation,
    164
children, 36–37
  in decision-making process,
    36–37
  names and addresses of, 110
  sick, guidelines for care of,
    164–66
  terminally ill, 161–66
Children's Blood Foundation,
    189
Church of Religious Science,
    200
citizenship papers, 109
City of Hope, 183, 190
Cobley's Anemia Foundation,
    189
columbarium, 136
Commerce Department, U.S.,
    109
Committee for Freedom of
    Choice in Cancer Therapy,
    196
Committee to Combat
    Huntington's Disease, 184
communication:
  with doctors, 31–32, 69–74,
    79–80
  of effects of medication,
    31–32
  home care and, 89
  illusion of, 70–71, 73
  among patients, care-givers
    and doctors, 70–71
computerized referral donor
    programs, 124–26
Concerned Relatives of Nursing
    Home Patients, 191–92
consumer credit counselors, 119
Continental Associations of

Funeral & Memorial
    Societies, 137, 200
contracts, 110
convalescent homes, *see* nursing
    homes
Cortner, Jean A., 190
cosmetology, 132–33
Council of Teaching Hospitals,
    186
County Health Services, 89
couples, *see* nontraditional
    couples
credit, 120–21
credit cards, 112
credit counselors, 119
credit-life insurance, 130
cremation, 111, 135–36
Cystic Fibrosis Center, 193

death benefits, 128–29
debts, 121–22
decision-making:
  children in, 36–37
  physical changes and, 29
  resistance to, by terminally
    ill, 34–35
  during shock, 18
  stress and, 50–52
denial, 18–19
Department of Family Life, 200
diabetes, 188
diagnosis, drug-related
    grouping in, 86
"Dial-a-Prayer," 200
divorce papers, 110
doctors, 67–74
  communication with, 31–32,
    69–74, 79–80
  expectations and, 70
  faith in, 68
  professional perspective vs.
    indifference of, 69
  questions for, 71–73
  selection of, 68–69
Do It Now Foundation, 182
Donor Registration Form, 198
DRG (diagnosis-related
    grouping), 86

Dysautonomia Foundation, 184
Dystonia Foundation, 184

elderly, 153–60
    resource-reference material
        for, 159–60
embalming, 132–33
emotions, 17–26
    blocking of, 18, 21, 24
    guidelines for dealing with,
        24–26
    see also specific emotions
employee benefits, 129
Epilepsy Foundation of
    America, 193
Episcopalian churches, 109
Equinox Institute, 201
euthanasia, 21–22, 128, 170
Eye Bank for Sight Restoration,
    198

Family Life Bureau, 200
Family Service Association of
    America, 200
finances, 117–22
    assets, 118
    expenses, 118–19
    getting help with, 35–36,
        119
    law, 120
free-standing hospice, 96
Friedreich's Ataxia Group in
    America, 184
friends, 55–63
    acquaintances vs., 40–41
    asking for help from, 41–42
    in household finances,
        35–36
    stress relieved by, 48–50
    supportive, 58–59
Funeral Director's Association,
    134
funerals, 131–38
    checklists for, 136–37
    cost of, 131–32
    optional expenses, 132
    professional services, 132

Garfield, Charles, 194
Gay and Lesbian Advocates and
    Defenders, 196
Gay Medical Association, 197
Gay Men's Health Crisis
    (GMHC), 150, 151–52, 197
Gay Men's Health Crisis
    Hotline, 196
Gay Rights National Lobby,
    149
gay rights organizations, 149
gays, 148–49
Georgia Warm Springs
    Foundation, 184–85
Gerontological Society, 159,
    200
gifts:
    for care-givers, 60–61
    for terminially ill persons,
        142–43
Gonzales, Frederico, 197
grave markers, 136
Gray Panthers, 159
grieving:
    healing and, 168
    pre-death, 24, 33
guilt, 10, 19–20, 165–66

hallucinations, 31, 32–33
Health, Education and Welfare
    Department, 102, 118
Health and Human Services
    Department, U.S., 101, 152,
        196
health insurance, 76–77, 118,
    128–29, 153–54
Health Maintenance
    Organizations (HMOs), 97
Heart Disease Research
    Foundation, 194
heart diseases, 194
helper groups, 61
Hemlock Society, 170, 187
hemodialysis, 186
hemophilia, 186, 190
hemorrhagia of newborn, 190
Herpetics Engaged in Living
    Productively (HELP), 192

215

Hill-Burton Act (1946), 77, 101
home care, 60, 88–95
    comunication and, 89
    cost of, 89–90
    equipment for, 93–95
    preparation for, 88, 92
    routine in, 92–93
Home-Care Hospice Programs,
    97
homophobia, 151, 152
hospices, 92, 96–100
    for AIDS victims, 149
    criteria and standards for,
        98–99
    with extended care facilities,
        97
    free-standing, 96
    hospital-affiliated,
        free-standing, 96
    hospital-based, 96–97
    teams in, 97, 99
hospital bills, 76–77, 101–2
hospitals, 75–81
    accounting department of, 76,
        80–81
    child care in, 80
    complaints about, 77–81
    cost of, 118
    information on, 79
    organization of, 75–76
    privacy in, 78
    regulations of, 77, 101
    support from staff of, 73–74
    visitors in, 77–78
household help, 37–38
Human Resources Department,
    77, 107
Human Services Department,
    63
Human Unity Councils, 200
Huntington's disease, 184, 185

impotence, 29–30
Independent Citizens Research
    Foundation for the Study of
    Degenerative Diseases, 188
indifference, 33–34
insurance, 23, 110

health, 76–77, 118, 128–29,
    153–54
life, 110, 129–30
Medicaid, 85, 86, 111, 158,
    192
Medicare, 85, 86, 154, 158,
    192
internal organs, artificial, 199
International Association of
    Cancer Victims and
    Friends, 195
International Bundle Branch
    Block Association, 194
International Foundation for
    Cancer Research, 195
International Naturopathic
    Association, 183
International Order of the
    Golden Rule, 138
intestate, dying, 116–17
IRAs (Individual Retirement
    Accounts), 110

job titles, 110
joint ownership, 112–13
Justice Department, Calif., 156

Keogh accounts, 110
Kubler-Ross, Elizabeth, 20, 73

Last Will and Testament, 117
    sample form, 173–74
lawyers, *see* attorneys
Legal Aid Society, 107, 117,
    148, 154
Legal Services for the Elderly
    Poor, 160
lesbians, 148–49
Letters of Intent, 34, 111, 122,
    123–24, 171–72
leukemia, 186–87, 189
Leukemia Society of America,
    186
life insurance, 110, 129–30
Limited Power of Attorney,
    127
Lion's Sight Foundation, Inc.,
    198

Living Bank, 124–26, 136, 198
Living Trusts, 122–23
Living Wills, 22, 51, 79, 111, 126–28
sample form, 170
Lou Gehrig's disease, 184, 185
Lupus Erythematosus, 182

Make Today Count, 150, 197
Mann, Thomas, 9
marriage certificates, 109
mausoleums, 135
Medicaid, 85, 86, 111, 158, 192
Medical Health Association, 193
Medical Power of Attorney, 127
Medicare, 85, 86, 154, 158, 192
medication:
behavior and, 21
communicating effects of, 31–32, 69–70
cost of, 118
improper, 30–32
for shock, 18
memorials, 131–38
Mental Health Materials Center, 193
military discharge papers, 110
military records, 109
Miller, Alan V., 197
miracle cures, 18–19
Mitford, Jessica, 138
monuments, 136
Motor Vehicle Department, 114
multi-infarct dementia, 187
multiple sclerosis, 191
Muscular Dystrophy Association, 185
mutual funds, 111
Myasthenia Gravis Foundation, 185

National ALS Foundation, 185
National Association for Spanish-Speaking Elderly, 159
National Association of Area Agencies on Aging, 160
National Association of

Children's Hospitals and Related Institutes, 186
National Association of Patients on Hemodialysis, 186
National Cancer Programs, 201
National Center of Black Aged, 159
National Committee for Research in Neurological and Communicative Disorders, 185
National Committee on Treatment of Intractable Pain, 192
National Continuing Care Directory, 160
National Council of Family Relations, 200
National Council of Senior Citizens, 159
National Council on Aging, 159, 201
National Easter Seal Society for Crippled Children and Adults, 193
National Gay Task Force, 152, 196
National Genetic Foundation, 193
National Hemophilia Foundation, 186
National Hospice Organization, 100, 192
National Huntington's Disease Association, 185
National Indian Council on Aging, Inc., 159
National Jewish Hospital/National Asthma Center, 190
National Kidney Foundation, 186
National Leukemia Association, 186–87
National Library of Medicine, 198
National Lupus Erythematosus Foundation, 182

National Multiple Sclerosis Society, 191
National Parkinson Foundation, 191
National Rare Blood Club, 187
National Rey's Syndrome Foundation, 190–91
National Senior Citizens Law Center, 160
National Spinal Cord Injury Foundation, 190
National Tay-Sachs and Allied Diseases Association, 193–94
Natural Death Act, 126
New York Hospital–Cornell Medical Center, 189–90
next of kin, 148
nightmares, 37
"No Code," 22, 78–79, 127–28
nontraditional couples, 147–52
  Agreement to Live Together, sample form, 176–78
  family problems of, 149
  legal relationship of, 147
notices of death, 136
NRTA/AARP (National Retired Teachers Association for Retired People), 159
nursing homes, 82–87
  in California, 154–57
  checking reputations of, 85–86
  costs of, 84–85
  director of, 84
  kitchen of, 84
  patients in, 83
  recreation in, 85
  regulations for, 154–56
  smell of, 83

On Death and Dying (Kübler-Ross), 20
One/Fourth, The Alliance for Cancer Patients and Their Families, 195
organ donor forms, 111
organ donor programs, 124–26, 136, 148, 198–99

palliative care, 97, 98
paranoia, 31
Parkinson Disease Foundation, 191
Parkinson's disease, 183, 191
partnership papers, 111
Patient Representatives, 77, 80
personal reference files, 111–12
pet car, 59
phone calls, 62, 141
plant care, 59
power of attorney, 51, 111
  Medical (Limited), 127
  sample form, 172–73
  Unlimited, sample form, 174–76
"Prayer for Serenity," 45
pre-death grieving, 24
  withdrawal as, 33

Reach for Recovery, 195
Reader's Digest, 52
record keeping, 114–16
Records Departments, city, county or state, 109
Red Cross, 56, 192
Rey's syndrome, 190–91
right-to-die laws, 127

safety deposit boxes, 110, 111, 122
Saint Jude Children's Research Hospital, 188
Salvation Army, 56
sample forms, 169–78
savings accounts, 110
savings certificates, 111
school records, 109
second opinions, 69, 162
self-pity, 38
sexual needs, of terminally ill patient, 29–30
Shanti, 149, 150, 194
shock, 17–18
  medication for, 18
shopping, 61–62
sickle cell anemia, 190
sick rooms, emotional responses to, 22–23

smoking, 40
Social Security, 153–54
  death benefits from, 128–29
social security number, 110
social service workers, 37–38
Society for the Right to Die,
  127, 170, 187
Society of Compassionate
  Friends, 201
sorrow, 24
Spiritual Frontiers Fellowship
  (SFF), 199
spiritual healing, 43, 45, 52–54,
  199–200
"Standards of a Hospice
  Program of Care, The," 98
State Office on Aging, 201
stock options, 110
stoicism, 44
stress, 17, 43–54
  caffeine and, 46–47
  controlling of, 43–53
  decision-making and, 50–52
  friends' role in relief of,
    48–50
  illness and, 46
  relieving of, 45–52
  religion and, 52–54
  symptoms of, 43–44
  treatment for, 45
Sunshine Foundation, 189
support groups, 56–58, 182–201
  after death, 167–68
support systems, 55–63
  community groups as, 56–58
  for families with terminally
    ill children, 163–64
  spiritual, 55–56
  see also care-givers; friends;
    household help
surviving spouse:
  finances handled by, 35–36
  independence of, 37
  responsibilities of, 38
  support systems for, see
    support systems
survivorship, 112–13

tax accountants, 107
tax deductions, 114–15
taxes, 121
  keeping records and, 114–16
tax forms, 110
terminally ill:
  babying of, 145–46
  behavior changes in, 20–21
  changes in personality of,
    30–33
  children, 161–66
  decision-making of, 34–35
  diet of, 40
  doctor's orders and, 39–40
  egocentrism of, 38–39
  environmental changes and,
    29, 141–42
  family of, 110
  gifts for, 142–43
  hope of, 146
  mental attitude of, 19, 29, 34,
    38–40, 141–42, 146
  physical and sexual needs of,
    29–30
  records of, 108
  talking to, 143–46
  telling truth to, 73–74
  treatment resisted by, 19
  visits to, 32–33, 141–46,
    150–51
Texas Medical Center, 124
thalassemia, 190
therapy, sexual, 30
titles of ownership, 110
total patient care, see hospices
transferring of titles, 113–14
transplants, 124–26
treatment:
  alternatives to, 18–19
  cost of, 119
  resistance to, 19
  side-effects of, 28

Understanding the New
  California Nursing Home
  Law (Younger), 156
Uniform Anatomical Gift Act,
  124, 198

Uniform Donor Card, 198
union benefits, 110
United Cancer Council, 195
United Cerebral Palsy
　Association, 193
United Osomy Association, 192
United Parkinson Foundation,
　191
United Way, 63
Unity, 199
Urban Elderly Coalition, 160
urns, 135–36
USC-LA County Medical Center,
　183
utilities, 112

Variety Clubs International,
　189
Very Important Papers, 105–30

veteran's benefits, 129
Visiting Nurses Association
　(VNA), 56, 88, 89, 92, 97
visits, 32–33, 141–46
　to elderly patients, 157
　with mutual friends, 142
　timing of, 142

Widow to Widow Program,
　201
wills, 105–6, 111, 116–17, 148
　Letters of Intent as, 123
　Living Trusts as, 122
　writing of, 51–52
withdrawal, 33
writing letters, 62
W-2 forms, 110

Younger, Euell J., 156